The *New* Diabetes Prescription

The Diet, Exercise,
and Mindset Revolution

AARON SNYDER

The New Diabetes Prescription: The Diet, Exercise, and Mindset Revolution

Published by:
Creative Arts Press, LLC
1385 Caminito Arriata
La Jolla, CA 92037

For orders, please visit our website:
http://www.TheNewDiabetesPrescription.com

First Edition
Designed by Gwyn Kennedy Snider
Photographs by Deborah Shields

ISBN: 978-0-9825441-2-9

WARNING – DISCLAIMER: Aaron Snyder is not a licensed physician and the statements regarding supplements in this book have not been reviewed by the FDA. The term "cure" when used throughout the book is used as a synonym for controlling blood sugar. Further, controlling blood sugar, defined by maintaining it within the range of 70 to 120 mg/dl for a given period of time, is not intended in any way to mean the same thing as curing type II diabetes. Further no other phrase, supplement, or general advice in this book is intended to portray the ability to "cure", treat, prevent, or diagnose any disease.

The information presented in this work is in no way intended as medical advice or as a substitute for medical treatment. This information should be used in conjunction with guidance and care of your physician, especially if you are taking medications, including diuretics or medications for blood pressure or diabetes. Consult your physician before embarking on any weight loss or exercise program or cutting your carbohydrates. The activities may be too strenuous or dangerous for some people and the reader(s) should consult a physician before engaging in them.

This book is sold with the understanding that the publisher and the author are not liable for the misconception or misuse of the information provided. Every effort has been made to make this book as complete and accurate as possible. The sole purpose is to educate. The author and publisher shall have neither liability nor responsibility to any person or entity with respect to any loss, damage, or injury caused or alleged to be caused directly or indirectly by the information contained in this book.

Mention of specific companies, organizations, or authorities in this book does not imply endorsement by the publisher, nor does mention of specific companies, organizations, or authorities imply that they endorse this book.

DEC 2010

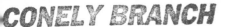

ACKNOWLEDGMENTS

To Antoinette Kuritz, for taking a chance on an unknown. For your guidance, persistence, and ingenious solutions to the countless problems that arise during the publishing process—thank you, thank you, thank you. To Dr. John Legler, who casually suggested that "I write a book about it." It was a suggestion we both know was quite premeditated. It's one of those sentences that change your life. To my father, David Snyder, who only once suggested that I was crazy for writing a book when I was laid off, and for his continued and unquestionable support from then on, including the laptop for Christmas. And to my mother, Marjorie Snyder, who has believed in me unconditionally since birth.

To my Aunt Lois and Uncle Frank, for teaching me the purpose of literature and writing over casual afternoon conversations – lessons that taught me more than years and years spent in English classes. You are both true teachers. To CH, for teaching me what she needed to teach me. I know who I am thanks to you.

To Rebecca Stern and Rich Kuritz, for such fantastic bookings while working around my horrid schedule. To Tim Johnson for top-notch website support and advice. Special thanks to Gwyn Kennedy Snider for designing the interior and exterior of this work and Deborah Shields for taking all the photos.

And finally, to everyone I have ever encountered who taught me something about human behavior, and to the countless people I will later realize I failed to acknowledge only after this goes to print – my thanks and apologies.

*This work is dedicated to my beloved Oksana,
the Light of my Life, without whom
none of this would have happened.
You are strong everywhere I am not.
Thank you for your patience, love, and support.
And to Alec, who sacrificed bedtime stories,
trips to Legoland, and days at the beach
without his consent so Papa RiRi could type
on his computer. For this, I am truly sorry.
I love you both.*

CONTENTS

It matters not how strait the gate,
How charged with punishments the scroll,
I am the master of my fate:
I am the captain of my soul.

Invictus, by William Ernest Henley

PREFACE

My life changed for the better the day I learned I was diabetic, the day I finally started dealing with my binge eating disorder, though it didn't feel that way then. No one ever forgets that day. It starts with shock and shifts into utter disbelief before ending in total confusion over the thousand facts you don't even know that you don't know.

I was diagnosed with type II diabetes on September 6, 2000 at age twenty-two. The meal that revealed my condition was a rare filet mignon paired with garlic mashed potatoes, buttered croissants, chocolate mousse, and Irish cream liqueur. My dinner companion, also a diabetic, decided this was the perfect opportunity to test what she had long suspected – that my blurry vision, fatigue, and frequent urinating were all classic signs of the disease. Using a single drop of my blood, extracted from her lancet, she then placed the drop on a little strip attached to her glucometer. The result only took thirty seconds, but it was the look on her face that told me what it meant. "OK," she said in a dead-pan tone that made the words seem to drop like cement bricks. She flashed me the screen. It read 211 mg/dl, a definitive sign of the disease. A subsequent visit to the doctor's office proved her suspicions and diagnosis correct.

I was in total shock. I had never had anything seriously wrong with me my entire life. Sure, I was overweight and ate a lot of junk food, but so did a lot of people. What was so different about me?

Type II doesn't usually hit until middle age, meaning my sedentary junk food lifestyle had put me ahead of schedule. If you have the genes to get diabetes, it certainly helps to eat junk food, not exercise, and gain weight. I was helping the disease in all three ways. With the doctor's diagnoses in hand, I was forced to admit that the late-night drive through runs and ice cream binges had taken their toll.

A few days later, as the news sunk in, I began to connect the dots between the other symptoms I'd been having. On several occasions, I had actually passed out after a particularly heavy doughnut or Oreo raid. Waking up, my hands would shake, my vision would blur, and I'd have little control over my bladder. Looking back, the diagnosis was obvious. But I didn't have the knowledge or experience to see it. In short, my body was giving me all the signs, but I wasn't getting the hint. To be honest, I don't think I wanted to.

By the time I was nineteen, I'd gone from overweight to normal weight and back several times. From ages six through eleven, I was consistently thirty pounds over what was considered healthy for my age. That heaviness affected everything in my life. Already a reserved child, I became the opposite of athletic, favoring TV and Legos over soccer and baseball. So I was continually placed in a "special" physical education class, usually reserved for the mentally and physically handicapped. Later, puberty took some weight off, but that was short lived; repeated binging packed it back on. By eighteen, I was 215 pounds on a 5'5" frame. Now I know that insulin surges from my as-yet unknown diabetes were helping my weight gain. But I also know that my overeating was the root cause of the problem.

It was common for me to eat four or five candy bars after a filling meal. I routinely downed entire cartons of ice cream when nervous, usually over a test. In high school, my nickname was "Bagel Boy," since I could easily go through a whole bag of bagels in one day. In short, I was a big emotional eater. I also didn't know that candy bars and bagels were exacerbating a condition in my body that would eventually lead to the sixth-deadliest and most costly disease in the United States.

My friend's amateur diagnosis that September night was my wakeup call. I was faced with a hard truth: abusing my body with junk food had a price, and that price could have been my life. I had to change, but I didn't know how. What I did know was what I wanted. I wanted to lose weight, and master my emotional eating. I wanted to take control of my life. To be honest, I failed at my first 1,000 attempts to change. It was years before I finally succeeded.

But when I finally did. . .

Today, in my thirties, I maintain a weight of around 155 pounds and have less than 8% body fat. My blood sugar is tightly controlled, and my cholesterol and blood pressure are close to perfect. It's not my superb genes that are responsible for this success. It's not a daily ten-mile run, or a cabbage soup and grapefruit diet, or a steady round of fifteen different medications. I don't exercise every day, and I can't remember the last time I went to bed hungry.

I do remember the pumpkin pie and ice cream I ate last Thanksgiving, and the cheesecake I had for my birthday two weeks before that. I remember that my last doctor's check-up showed my feet, eyes, heart, and kidneys were all perfectly healthy. I now have energy all day thanks to stable blood sugar. I can look at my life and see the control I have...

Changing my body started with changing my eating habits. Changing those habits started with changing my thinking. And it took me years. Not because the information wasn't out there. Not because there was too much of it. My transformation took so long because despite the number of books on the subject, and no matter how hard I looked, I couldn't find just one book that I thought was telling me the truth. Or the whole story. Every book told me that I needed to lose weight to control my blood sugar, but could I successfully stop weight gain when many of the medications that treat diabetes *make weight loss harder*? Likewise, blood pressure and cholesterol are better controlled through weight loss, and I had several diabetic friends on meds that treat those conditions. Could they lose enough weight to get off their blood pressure and cholesterol meds that were *also* causing weight gain? This was just the start of a whole host of other questions. How do you find the energy to exercise when you're so exhausted that you can barely make it home from work? How do you recover from hypoglycemia without eating your weight in cookies? How do you keep away from those cookies when you've had another wretched day? Forget how readily available junk food is.

How do you eat right when even too much *fruit* is bad for you?

These challenges are unique to diabetics. They are unique to those of us that live this life.

I wasn't finding the answers I needed in any of the books I read. So I found my own way. And I'd like to share it.

The ultimate goal of this book is to teach you how to control diabetes through diet, exercise, and lifestyle *first*, and medications *second*.

That's the opposite approach many people take. First, they take the doctor's prescriptions, and *maybe then* attempt to eat better and exercise. But consider that weight loss effectively controls diabetes while many medications for diabetes make weight loss harder by how they control blood sugar. So by doing everything *you* can to control blood sugar, and only resorting to medication if absolutely necessary, you accelerate weight loss, which lowers blood sugar while avoiding side effects like fatigue. It doesn't mean you'll never eat pizza again. It doesn't mean you can stop taking all your meds and fire your doctor. It doesn't mean you won't slip up. It just means that you'll be controlling this disease and all its complications as much as possible through diet, exercise, and supplements. You'll only have to take the meds that are absolutely necessary.

I will teach you how to exercise no matter what your fitness level, and I'll eliminate time as the reason you don't exercise. I will never ask a lot of time from you. I will ask you for your *focus* in that time. You'll be able to live a life that makes you healthier, not sicker.

It's easier than you think. It's not a pipe dream. It's not unrealistic.

You may be surprised that lack of knowledge is not the true stumbling block on the path to healing. Even after I learned to control my blood sugar, the emotional eater within still binged. And when I learned to deal with my emotions, I still found myself in relationships with others who wanted to binge, using those relationships as an excuse.

Once I did, and I became consistent enough with exercising and eating well to reap the benefits, my blood sugar finally came under control.

> I learned while trying to heal that the greatest obstacle to healing was *me*. I wasn't really able to follow my own program until I fixed my relationship with myself and everyone else.

And now it's time for you to do the same.

So what do you do next? Unlike what you might expect, I won't ask you to give up a food or food group. From what you learn, you may decide that there's a better time to eat some foods, to opt for a lower carbohydrate version, or to simply consume less of it. You have your own preferences and habits, and your "sinful" foods are here to stay in your diabetic eating style. You just have to find a healthy way to deal with them. For example, there is always a time for dessert, even when your stomach is flat and you flaunt a six-pack year round. As a fellow diabetic for whom too much dessert too often has grave consequences, hear me. There is always a time for dessert.

I'm going to be giving you reams of information, advice, and instructions. It will be up to you to decide whether applying this newfound knowledge is worth regaining your health and, in the process, losing 20, 50, or even 100 pounds. The rewards, however, are far greater than simple weight loss. It's the improved quality of life and the boost in self-esteem. It's the increased energy, the improved relationships, and the ability to actually be there for loved ones. It's knowing that you're giving yourself the chance to live a long life and to die of natural causes.

These are the reasons to change.

I will be asking you to examine some tough questions. I'll ask you to look inside yourself and identify why you want that change. Every time you crawl out of bed in the morning to exercise, and every time you prepare healthy meals in advance, I'll ask why you're doing it. I want you to know your own reasons, so you can see exactly why it's all worth it.

The Twelve New Diabetes Prescriptions

So how did I do it? Was it all low fat, low carb, or vegan food? Was it eating tofu and bean sprouts sprinkled with wheat germ in a cup of urine? Of course not! I looked at my life, figured out what worked and what didn't, and built twelve natural "prescriptions" for myself. These twelve prescriptions won't put a pound on you. They'll never make you tired, and they won't empty your pocketbook. They have no side effects except for weight loss, increased energy, and peace of mind. And they do what no medication in the world could do: they give you control over the hand that fate dealt you. They give you a way to "cure" yourself of that diabetic lifestyle.

> **These twelve prescriptions give you control over the hand that fate dealt you.**

- First Prescription: Be accountable and take control
- Second Prescription: Control emotional eating to control blood sugar
- Third Prescription: Change the stress, or change your response
- Fourth Prescription: Exercise is the best medication
- Fifth Prescription: Follow a low-carbohydrate diet most of the time

- Sixth Prescription: Eat the foods that heal, avoid the foods that kill
- Seventh Prescription: Choose your carbs wisely
- Eighth Prescription: Know what, when, and how much to eat
- Ninth Prescription: Know your diabetic complications, their medications, and your alternatives
- Tenth Prescription: Find healthy recipes that taste better than your unhealthy favorites
- Eleventh Prescription: When you feel like cheating, remember why you want to be healthy
- Twelfth Prescription: Put it together, write it down, and follow through

Prescribing the Maximum Dosage Rather Than the Minimum

If you take all twelve new prescriptions to heart and dedicate yourself 100%, you'll completely reverse the cause of your diabetes: inactivity, weight gain, and too many of the wrong foods. You'll get your blood sugar and diabetic complications under total control using as few medications as possible, if any. If you still need medications, they'll only be serving to reinforce your own efforts. They will no longer control your life. As you move through the program, you'll see continued and escalated progress. You'll lose weight faster. You'll get your energy back. You'll sleep better. You'll worry less about your future. You'll feel less anxious, because you'll know that this time you're really doing everything you can.

Before we jump into details about the twelve prescriptions, I must ask you one question. It's the most important question you'll ever answer, because it contains the secret to your weight loss, future health, and longevity.

Why do you want to change?

Look inside yourself and answer – what would be the best thing about being healthy again? What is it about slimming down and having energy that would give you peace of mind? What thoughts and feelings ring true enough to you that you'll be motivated to wake up earlier and exercise, or work out when you've had a long and tiring day? Why do you love yourself enough that you would choose to forgo a second serving of dessert? Why would you be willing to bring your own food when everyone else is eating pizza? In short, why is it all worth it? Think of your answer and write it down. Paste it on your fridge. Think about it while you read this book. In the end, it's the only reason you'll do a single thing I ask.

Aaron Snyder
San Diego, CA
May 2010

The New Diabetes Prescription

The Diet, Exercise, and Mindset Revolution

*"The ultimate goal of this book is to teach you how to control diabetes through diet, exercise, and lifestyle **first**, and medications **second**."*

INTRODUCTION

The preferred route for most diabetics is to find a doctor we trust and follow his or her instructions to the letter. The doctor, we surmise, knows what diabetes is, how to best treat it, what we really need. But with that mindset, we are once again playing into what got us here in the first place; we are abrogating our personal responsibility for our own health.

In living *The New Diabetes Prescription*, I took responsibility for my health. In writing *The New Diabetes Prescription*, I am sharing with you what I did that worked so that you have a roadmap for stepping into responsibility for *your* health.

It is easy to vest this responsibility in our doctors. But is it best?

In learning the root causes of diabetes, the alternative treatments, the supplements that can keep us from indulging in the behaviors that caused our diabetes in the first place, we become proactive. And while all the details may at times seem a bit overwhelming, and while the learning curve may take some time, once you vest yourself with control over this disease, you will find that not just your physical well-being but your emotional and spiritual health will improve as well.

This book is full of information. Don't skip any of it. It is necessary for you to understand the physical and psychological reasons for your diabetes, to understand how your body works, and to understand fully what steps you can take to mitigate your diabetes if you are to take control.

At the end of the book I have simplified the information into menu suggestions along with a list of supplements to take, when to take them, and how much to take; the information is synthesized for your use. But again, read through it all.

Much of this information will either be new to you or it will be more detailed than you are used to getting. It might take time to digest. Read it, reread it, and make it your own. All of it will become integral to the journey on which you are about to embark, a journey to better health, and, as a result, an overall better life. *The New Diabetes Prescription* makes sense. It worked for me. It will work for you.

"It's time to stop depending on someone—or something—else to save you. The sooner you can accept this, the sooner you can change."

1

THE FIRST PRESCRIPTION

Be Accountable and Take Control

*I*t's the twenty-first century, and we don't yet have a pill that will let you eat whatever you want and still lose weight. We don't have a pill that "cures" diabetes. Gastric bypass is the new trend to treat diabetes if you're heavy enough. It works by making you throw up if you eat too much, but that's really the only thing it accomplishes. I personally know of a woman who lost more than 100 pounds over two years after gastric bypass, but who has gained back more than half of that in the five years since. The reason is simple: she never really developed new eating habits. Her old behaviors returned as her stomach stretched back out.

> **It's time to stop depending on someone – or something – else to save you. The sooner you can accept this, the sooner you can change.**

The First Prescription will teach you all about diabetes. It will tell you how you got here, and how to become accountable for your own health. Controlling diabetes does not end with a doctor's prescription. This isn't a cold you're dealing with; it's one of the most deadly diseases in the world. You can't just take the pills and shots and wait for it to get better. Of the top six deadliest diseases, this one is the most manageable in your hands. Its improvement depends mostly on things you control, like diet and exercise. With a blood sugar monitor, you get immediate feedback on whether what you're doing is working or not. If your blood sugar goes up over time, the answer is simple: you did something to cause that. On the other hand, if your blood sugar goes down, you did something to cause *that*. The power to heal is in your hands. But so is the responsibility. Accept that, and let's move toward healing.

Diabetes Is <u>NOT</u> Going Away

> **The National Institutes of Health estimates there are over 24 million Americans with diabetes today, 25% of whom don't even know they have it. Another 57 million have pre-diabetes.[1] The CDC estimates one in three Americans born after 2000 will get diabetes in their lifetime.[4-5] They are calling it an epidemic.[2]**

Around the world, there are over 170 million diabetics, a number expected to double by 2030.[3] Ninety percent of those are type II diabetics while the other 10 percent are type I's and those with less common forms like cystic fibrosis-related diabetes (CFRD), maturity onset diabetes of the youth (MODY), and gestational diabetes. While gestational diabetes often clears up after giving birth, the mother is at greater risk of getting type II diabetes if the newborn baby weighed more than 9 pounds.

All forms of diabetes have one thing in common, *high blood sugar* or hyperglycemia. That's how diabetics get those famous symptoms of frequent urination, thirst, excessive hunger, fatigue, and blurry vision. While a non-diabetic's blood sugar nearly always stays within the range of 70 to 120 milligrams of glucose per deciliter of blood (mg/dl), a diabetic's can swing upwards to 200, 300, or even 500 mg/dl! At that level of blood sugar, the level of toxins in the blood and dehydration can be fatal.

Low blood sugar, or hypoglycemia, can also occur from taking medications for diabetes or from a diabetic's own erratic blood sugar swings. Symptoms include rapid heartbeat, profuse sweating, confusion, irritability, and excessive hunger, in particular for sweets. While hypoglycemia does not technically occur until blood sugar dips below 70 mg/dl, these symptoms can be felt when blood sugar drops suddenly, such as from 180 mg/dl to 120 mg/dl in a very short amount of time. Extremely low blood sugar will starve the brain of glucose. And yes, just as with *hyper*glycemia, *hypo*glycemia can be fatal.

> **Type I diabetics will need insulin for the rest of their lives. Type II diabetes is a different story.**

While the symptoms for high blood sugar remain the same in all diabetics, how those symptoms appear depends on the kind of diabetes. In type I diabetes, an autoimmune disorder kills off the part of the pancreas that makes insulin, the hormone that takes glucose from the blood and sticks it in our cells. This usually happens in early childhood or adolescence, which is why type I diabetes was once also known as child-onset diabetes. However, since over 25 percent of all newly diagnosed diabetics under twenty years old are of the type II variety, and 7% of all children in America are pre-diabetic[1], that definition no longer applies.

Type I diabetics will need insulin for the rest of their lives. This book can help them need less of it and help them control complications, but they must have that insulin to survive.

Type II diabetes was once also known as adult-onset diabetes, but as just mentioned, the explosion in the number of kids getting it has made that definition obsolete. Here, blood sugar rises due to insulin resistance, a direct cause of obesity, inactivity, and overeating. Since the cells cannot take up insulin, glucose remains in the blood. Weight control is considered the most effective "cure" for type II diabetes, but the predisposition to develop insulin resistance will always be there. Therefore, controlling type II diabetes is a lifelong affair.

Pre-diabetes is an early form of type II diabetes. It goes by many other names like Syndrome "X," metabolic syndrome, impaired fasting glucose (IGF), and impaired glucose tolerance (IGT). Regardless, they all mean the same thing—insulin resistance has set in, and blood sugar levels are abnormal, but not yet to the point of qualifying as diabetic.

It is extremely common for both diabetics and pre-diabetics to have a family history of diabetes. They're often overweight and usually have high cholesterol and high blood pressure when diagnosed. Dark patches may appear on their skin called acanthosis nigricans, caused by high blood sugar. There is often a parent or sibling also with type II diabetes. In my case, my great-grandmother, grandfather, mother, and I all have it.

The terms type I and type II diabetic are sometimes replaced with insulin dependent diabetes mellitus (IDDM) for the type I's and non-insulin dependent diabetes mellitus (NIDDM) for the type II's. That preference is made based on the number of type I's who have developed insulin resistance and the number of type II's whose diabetes is so far gone that they now need insulin. In this book, I will simply refer to type II diabetes as diabetes, and I make no distinction as to whether the said diabetic is or is not on insulin.

From here on out, I will be referring only to type II diabetes, but make no mistake that all forms of diabetes can be helped by this book. The key difference is that while it is possible for type II diabetics to control their disease without medication, all type I's, most cystic fibrosis-related diabetics, and a few MODYs will need their insulin.

How Diabetes Is Diagnosed

The World Health Organization has established the diagnoses for diabetes in one of three ways:

1) A fasting blood sugar of 126 mg/dl or more.

2) A glycated hemoglobin (HbA1c) of 6.0% or higher. This is basically a three-month average measurement of your blood sugar. An A1c of more than 6.0% means that your blood sugar measurements have been consistently greater than 120 mg/dl for more than three months. A 1.0% increase or decrease in A1c is roughly equivalent to a 30 mg/dl increase or decrease in blood sugar.

3) Two random blood sugar readings of 200 mg/dl or more on separate occasions, with at least a few of the classic symptoms of diabetes such as thirst, frequent urination, or fatigue.

Pre-diabetes is defined as having a fasting blood sugar between 100 mg/dl and 125 mg/dl, or a postprandial (after eating) blood sugar of greater than 140 mg/dl. If left unchecked, most cases of pre-diabetes will progress to full-blown diabetes. Regardless, pre-diabetics run a greater than normal risk of acquiring all complications of diabetes, including stroke, heart attack, blindness, kidney failure, neuropathy, and amputations[6].

How Diabetes Develops and Causes Weight Gain

Insulin resistance is the trademark of type II diabetes. Insulin is excreted by the pancreas after the first bite of food, and later on in boluses, or little squirts, to keep blood sugar stable. Among the three major nutrients, carbohydrates require far more insulin to process than protein or fat. In fact, fat eaten without any carbohydrates barely requires any insulin at all. To summarize, you eat, glucose is processed, and insulin transports that glucose to your cells so they can eat. Insulin resistance requires more insulin than normal to make that whole process work.

The amount of insulin needed to process a gram of glucose into your cells is not fixed. It varies from person to person, and even hour to hour! People who need very little insulin to process their food are called insulin sensitive. Insulin sensitivity is increased with exercise, eating healthy, having more muscle, and keeping lean. In contrast, type II diabetics are insulin resistant because they may need up to four or more times the amount of insulin of a normal individual to process their food. Insulin resistance is increased through not exercising, eating a diet high in refined sugars and fats, and as a consequence, gaining too much body fat. This creates huge surpluses in glucose that must be cleared from the blood by huge surpluses in insulin.

Developing insulin resistance to the level of diabetic or pre-diabetic takes years, but the causes can be attributed to just three factors: excess sugar, insulin, and fat in the blood.

Excess blood sugar causes glycation, the unintended bonding of sugar with proteins and lipids. This haphazard bonding creates what are known as advanced glycation end products (AGEs) and free radicals that wreak all sorts of havoc in the body, leading to diabetes and a host of other degenerative diseases. AGEs damage the beta cells, causing even higher blood sugar and insulin resistance. They damage the endothelial lining of the blood vessels, causing plaque to form in the larger arteries. This stiffens the arteries, causing atherosclerosis, putting you at risk of a heart attack or stroke. Glycation also stiffens the collagen in blood vessels, increasing blood pressure and these risks even further. And since glycated cells are cleared very slowly from the body, the kidneys, eyes, nerves, and DNA are damaged over time.

Interestingly, not all forms of sugar cause the same degree of glycation. Fructose found in fruit, fruit juice, and soda, and galactose--found in dairy products--are far more glycating than straight glucose. In fact, fructose causes ten times the glycation compared to glucose. It shouldn't be surprising then that sodas and other products containing high fructose corn syrup are linked to diabetes.

Excess insulin in the blood causes insulin resistance by destroying the GLUT4 insulin receptors on the exterior of cells. These receptors actually move glucose into cells without the help of insulin. Losing your GLUT4 receptors means even less glucose can get into the cells, forcing the body to produce even more insulin. With each increase in insulin, more insulin receptors are damaged, and the process ensues. Glucose that cannot enter the muscle cells will be diverted to the fat cells, making them larger. Further, all that extra insulin severely blocks hormone-sensitive lipase (HSL), the enzyme that breaks down body fat. So the more insulin circulating through your system, the more fat you'll gain, especially in your gut.

Have you ever noticed people who are stressed, have heart problems, or have diabetes tend to carry most of their fat around their middle? Diabetics and pre-diabetics often have an "apple-shaped" build, where fat is concentrated in the abdomen rather than throughout the entire body. There is a very good reason for this. It's the center of your body and home to a kind of fat that surrounds your internal organs, known as visceral fat. This special kind of abdominal fat is responsible for a pot belly. It's different from the fat you can pinch around your belly button, love handles, buttocks, or thighs – that is, fat just under the skin, dubbed subcutaneous fat.

Visceral fat is full of toxins and hormones that, due its close placement near internal organs, can be easily released directly into your bloodstream and liver.[13] Treating your blood stream like a sewer, the excess fat releases abnormal amounts of hormones and chemical messengers like cytokines that cause inflammation to your endothelial tissue, the thin lining around blood vessels that helps transport nutrients into cells.[19] These inflammatory markers also distort how insulin interacts with your fat and muscle tissue, further increasing insulin resistance. For this reason, visceral fat is regarded as a marker for cardiovascular disease and diabetes. Just having a large waist circumference greater than forty inches in men and thirty-five inches in women increases your likelihood of having a heart attack or stroke.

Visceral fat's close proximity to the liver also contributes to non-alcoholic fatty liver disease (NAFLD). The excess fat that's been created causes the liver to overproduce triglycerides, cholesterol, and even more blood sugar, exacerbating insulin resistance even further.

Once all these problems are in place, you still may not be a full blown diabetic. You may only be insulin resistant and overweight. The body is still putting up a fight against the invasion of excessively high blood sugar levels by manufacturing an army of insulin to clear it all from the blood. Unfortunately, it's a lot easier to create more glucose than it is to manufacture more and more insulin. After all, all it takes to make more glucose is another doughnut! If you continue to not exercise, and eat a diet high in calories from refined flour, sugar, and saturated fat, the loser will be your pancreas. It will fail to produce enough insulin to clear glucose from the blood, and your blood sugar will rise. The breakdown will happen in two stages, leading to diabetes.

Initially, your pancreas stops releasing the first big bolus of insulin with the first bite of food. It then tries to "make up" for the lack of first response by excreting too much insulin after the meal. With this response, your blood sugar swings wildly from too high to too low, causing hunger and carbohydrate cravings. Acting on those cravings only makes fat gain, insulin resistance, and pancreatic exhaustion worse.

In the second stage, the pancreas will stop producing and releasing as much insulin in boluses after eating. Blood sugar will invariably be high enough now to diagnose you with diabetes. The pancreas may completely stop producing insulin. You may need insulin injections, as much as four times the normal amount for someone of your weight, to counter the insulin resistance. This is the last stage in the development of type II diabetes.

How Stress Makes Diabetes Worse

Controlling diabetes is a day-to-day process, and stress can make every part of it harder. It makes blood sugar rise, elevates blood pressure and bad cholesterol, gives you cravings, and makes you gain weight. A lot of research has been done to link stress and diabetes, and the best we can say right now is that even if stress is not a cause of type II diabetes per se, it sure makes it worse.

Whenever your brain perceives a situation as stressful, whether that stress is mental, emotional, or physical, it immediately dips into your body's energy reserves. First, it signals the hypothalamus to release adrenal corticotrophin hormone (ACTH). ACTH then orders the adrenal glands to release adrenaline and cortisone, the two hormones responsible for mobilizing the body's energy stores.

From there, cortisone performs a very important job – it signals your liver to break down glycogen for extra energy as glucagon, insulin's opposite (because it raises instead of lowers blood sugar), orders the liver to do the same[7]. Glycogen is your glucose reserve, rather like a stored meal inside your body, and is created from carbohydrates and proteins.

As cortisone breaks down sugar, adrenaline and noradrenaline, known as catecholamines, get to work on breaking down fats. These hormones attach themselves to special adrenoreceptors outside of fat cells, known as beta receptors. By forming a metabolite known as cyclic adenosine monophosphate (cAMP), they activate hormone sensitive lipase to start breaking down fats so they can be burned in the mitochondria of your muscle cells. You now have a steady stream of ongoing energy for this "fight or flight" situation. Without these reserves, you'd be a sitting duck. This same process also occurs when you exercise, which is the perfect example of stress hormones doing their job properly. As you're about to read, that isn't the case when stress, fatigue, and overwork affect you day in and day out.

These are processes that the human body has perfected, since we respond to stress today the same way we did 20,000 years ago. Back then, the increased stress came from increased physical effort – the stress of running from a predator or hunting for your dinner. Unlike today, stress was related to extreme physical effort. In other words – *there was no fat gain* from the stress.

Evolution and civilized society have changed all that. Today, instead of responding to facing a wild boar like you might have 10,000 years ago, your body is faced with situations like your boss shouting at you. Your boss's angry facial expression, body movements, and loud voice all trigger the same feelings of anxiety and terror that an encounter with a saber-toothed tiger once did. Your body generates enough cortisone and adrenaline to take a life-threatening situation head on, but without the increased physical effort that should balance them. And there's an issue here: fixing an order with your biggest client will *never* match the physical strain of defending your children from a wild boar that just leapt into your cave. Herein lies the first problem. The stress you encounter today isn't a wild animal in the jungle. It's a wild animal in the office – your boss.

> **Your body has only one response to a threat; when faced with danger, it automatically preps you for the worst-case scenario. And then it becomes confused after going into a fight or flight mode with no need for physical activity.[8]**

That's a problem for the body – stress hormones are designed to meet extremely physically demanding tasks where the stakes are life or death. They're not designed to go off every time your boss takes out his marital problems on you. Your body prepped you for the worst the *moment* your boss opened up with "OH MY GOD! Why the *HELL* does page seven begin with…" As far as your hypothalamus was concerned, he was about to eat your firstborn. But you haven't sprinted for your life. You haven't defended your village from a pack of wild boars. Instead, you've been sitting at your computer, working via email and phone to fix the problem. Your brain is working furiously, but not your body.

The first time you confuse your body like this, it forgives you. Next time you need it, it will be right there with adrenaline and cortisone faster than you can say "you're fired." But after a while, your body starts to see that you're crying wolf and begins to call your bluff. It becomes conditioned to what it sees as your overreaction. Over-stimulated from the constant bombardment by stress hormones, the body starts to ignore their orders. This causes a major kink in the natural supply chain. The body begins to tell fat cells to ignore the order from adrenaline about releasing fat for energy. It understands that you're not going to do anything requiring major physical exertion, regardless of the alarms going off. When this blunting of fat release from adrenaline takes place, we say that your body has developed adrenaline resistance.[9-10] This is a major problem for anybody, but is especially hard on a diabetic trying to lose fat.

> **Adrenaline resistance means fat-loss resistance because it's literally the nudge on fat cells to release stored fat for fuel.**

It's highly involved in the fat-burning process, so any resistance to adrenaline will mean that cells *don't* release fat when they're told to. The problem is twofold: first, this means no energy boost. Second, it means no fat loss, which is particularly bad for diabetics since more body fat usually means higher blood sugar. Once the condition of adrenaline resistance is full blown, your body will become less willing to release stored fat when you exercise, diet, or get stressed. Overweight diabetics already have adrenaline resistance. In fact, they can be ten times less sensitive to the beta-2 adrenaline receptor than individuals of normal weight[24]. Fortunately, the more weight you lose, the less adrenaline resistant you may become[25].

Besides diabetics and the obese, anyone under severe stress from too much work, too little sleep, or an anxiety disorder is at risk for adrenaline resistance. The same is true for those with addictions to nicotine, amphetamines, caffeine, or alcohol. The ultimate risk is fat gain, mind-numbing fatigue, and high blood sugar. The solution is in this book.

Cortisone from Stress Makes You Fatter

When it comes to gaining weight because of stress, adrenaline resistance is only one of two devils. Remember all that cortisone your body released when your boss leapt into your office with his sharp teeth exposed and his chest puffed out? It stayed in your system long after the stress was over, and might still be circulating through your body up to three or four days later. At that point, the initial stress may have ended, but cortisone's ability to wreak havoc on your body is far from finished.[11]

When cortisone comes into contact with fat cells, particularly visceral fat, it sends a message that is the exact opposite of adrenaline – *store fat*. Visceral fat has four times more cortisone receptors than all other fat cells.[11] That means that these cells are receiving four times as many messages to store fat when the body is stressed. High cortisone levels also increase insulin resistance.[12] This is a major way stress contributes to diabetes. Cortisone is particularly damaging when diabetics eat unhealthily.

In a study done by Dr. John Yudkin, author of *Sweet & Dangerous*, healthy individuals who were fed a diet high in refined carbohydrates and sugar – the diet you would follow if you were *trying* to get type II diabetes – had elevated insulin levels and serum cortisone levels that were *300% to 400% higher than normal within two weeks*.[11] These were healthy people with normal blood sugar, under no significant stress. Their insulin levels spiked significantly, as did their cortisone levels, due to the consumption of highly processed foods. Imagine then how much fat you're putting on by eating that food when *you* are stressed.

> **If you've noticed weight gain in the belly when stressed, you've found its creator – chronically high cortisone levels and insulin resistance.**

How Diabetes Slows Metabolism and Causes Hunger

During the entire time that insulin resistance is developing in your body, a second problem, leptin resistance, is developing in your brain. Whether one causes the other or they both develop at the same time doesn't really matter so long as you understand how problems with leptin lead to excess hunger, weight gain, and a slow metabolism.

Leptin is a hormone excreted by your fat cells that controls body fat, hunger, and metabolism. This hormone is being produced inside your fat cells and orchestrates cortisone's and adrenaline's influence on your blood pressure, cholesterol, and blood sugar.[10] It is primarily increased either by having more body fat or after ingesting carbohydrates.

Over and over again each day your brain keeps tabs on how much fat you have by how much leptin comes knocking at its door. Since fatter people have more leptin, their brains expect more leptin to reach the hypothalamus, the part of your brain that regulates appetite and metabolism. Likewise, slimmer people's brains expect less leptin. Regardless of whether you're heavyset or slender, your brain is rigged to expect a certain amount of leptin from your fat cells. When you're eating enough calories to maintain your weight, the amount of leptin in your blood is highly correlated with how much body fat you have.

The hypothalamus controls a plethora of hormones and neurotransmitters responsible for increasing or decreasing both metabolism and hunger. If too much leptin reaches your hypothalamus, metabolism is increased and appetite is decreased. Unfortunately, if not enough leptin reaches the brain, metabolism is decreased and appetite is increased, particularly for foods loaded with high glycemic carbs and saturated fats. This is the reason you start to crave ice cream and pizza after a few days on a diet.

If you start a diet today, you will lose body fat as you cut calories. However, with less body fat comes less leptin production, and as a result, less leptin reaches the brain. As a consequence, appetite increases and metabolism decreases.

On the other hand, what happens if you overeat? You gain body fat. And with a rise in body fat comes a rise in leptin, and hence an increase in leptin levels. As a result, your appetite goes down and your metabolism goes up. This explains why you are not so hungry after a large meal, not only for the remainder of the day, but for the next few days. And this also explains why after the initial bloat and water gain wears off, you really don't gain much weight, if any, from *one* day of overfeeding. In one study, men who were massively overfed carbohydrates gained a little over five ounces of fat per day max[14].

Leptin is the scientific answer to what you've always known – dieting slows weight loss and provokes cravings, and overeating makes you disinterested in food for a few days afterward. Leptin also explains the set-point theory, or the reason that people tend to stay the same weight no matter what. The body is hard-wired for survival. It does not know you'd rather have six-pack abs than survive an ice age.

So far, you've read about leptin behaving normally in a non-diabetic. The more leptin in the brain, the faster your metabolism and the less your hunger will be. However, being diabetic makes leptin go haywire by causing leptin resistance.

For the same reasons that you previously learned you were resistant to the hormone insulin, you're also resistant to leptin. It's a direct consequence of excessive triglycerides created from excess body fat. Years of overeating highly processed foods in large quantities without exercise made you fatter, and the extra fat caused too much leptin to be excreted from your fat cells, bombarding your hypothalamus with too much of this hormone's message to elevate metabolism and shut off appetite, damaging the brain's leptin receptors in the process. As a result, those receptors became numb to leptin's orders. This is called leptin resistance. Just as you have a lot of insulin floating around your blood but little of it is reaching your cells, causing high blood sugar and weight gain, you have a lot of leptin in your blood with little of it reaching your brain, causing high appetite and slow metabolism.

Leptin resistance doesn't happen from just one big meal but from the leptin created by gaining lots of weight[17]. When researchers from Jefferson Medical College overfed eight healthy individuals around fifty-five calories for every pound they weighed over twelve hours, leptin rose 40% above normal and remained high until the next morning. The same researchers then overfed six normal men until they gained 10% of their body weight, and continued to overfeed them so they could maintain that weight for two weeks. By then, leptin had risen three-fold in all subjects, and their brains' response to leptin was directly correlated with the percentage of body fat gained[16]. So if you overeat in the short run, leptin will rise, elevate metabolism, but drop before it contributes to leptin resistance. However, if you gain a lot of fat, the extra leptin will certainly be enough to cause fat gain. Further, gaining muscle will add barely any leptin to your system. This study goes to show that you want enough leptin to keep metabolic rate high, but not so much that it causes weight gain.

Leptin resistance can also occur after years of abuse to your metabolism in one or more of the following ways[18]:

- A diet high in refined flour or high fructose corn syrup;
- Binge eating;
- Too strict a diet for too long or repetitive yo-yo dieting;
- Alcohol and amphetamine use, even excessive use of over-the-counter fat burners;
- Stress from food allergies, disease, lack of sleep, few rejuvenating activities, overwork, candida overgrowth, or emotional duress;

- Genetic predispositions to obesity, leptin resistance, and insulin resistance. Only around 5% of the obese population is truly genetically leptin deficient;
- Type II diabetes. Diabetics' swinging insulin levels can increase leptin, adding to resistance;
- Being overweight as a child.

All of these contribute to leptin resistance by damaging the hypothalamus's ability to detect the correct amount of leptin in the brain.

How Leptin Makes Food Cravings Worse

When a diabetic with insulin, leptin, and a certain degree of adrenaline resistance gets stressed, food cravings and overeating are almost inevitable. To understand why, you need to understand leptin's opposite, neuropeptide Y (NPY).

> **You can think of NPY and leptin as friends sitting on a teeter-totter – when one is high, the other is low. NPY is the chief hunger signal in your brain. When NPY is high, you're hungry. Stress elevates NPY and "overworks" either the left or right hemisphere of the brain. When the right brain is stressed, serotonin, the neurotransmitter that fights anxiety, depression, sadness, and carb cravings, gets depleted. NPY goes up and leptin goes down, all in all creating hunger from the high NPY and carb cravings from the low serotonin. In short, you'll get the munchies for cookies and ice cream.**

Subconsciously, the craving will serve to increase your sense of well-being, relieve some tension, and put you in a better mood by increasing serotonin. This won't increase your ability to do work, but will make you feel better about getting back to work. So you'll eat something a little sweet, serotonin and leptin rise, NPY falls, you feel better, and the crisis is over.

Likewise, when the left brain is stressed, dopamine, the neurotransmitter responsible for concentration, motivation, and drive, gets depleted. Dopamine is built from the amino acid tyrosine, found in all sources of protein, but abundant in cheese. Tyrosine is converted to levodopa via the enzyme tyrosine hydroxylase in the adrenal glands. Levodopa is then converted to dopamine in the brain while fat and salt increase the total amount of dopamine available.

> **So not surprisingly, a normally healthy but currently stressed-out individual with left brain stress will crave something high in protein, fat, and salt.**

Subconsciously, the stressed-out individual is looking for more motivation and focus to get back to work. Dopamine cravings are a desire to increase productivity, directly contributing to the bottom line, unlike serotonin cravings. After these individuals eat a cheeseburger, dopamine and leptin will rise, NPY will fall, and again, the crisis will end. But in a stressed-out diabetic, it's a different story.

In a leptin and adrenaline resistant diabetic, snacking on nachos or cheeseburgers will not produce enough levodopa in the adrenals due to adrenal fatigue. This means a dopamine deficiency will perpetuate and will continually drive more cravings for protein, fat, and salt. Secondly, the diabetics will produce leptin from their fat cells, but the leptin resistance will prevent enough of it from entering the brain. Therefore, NPY will stay elevated, leaving the hunger signal turned on. In this case, you will remain stressed, tired, and hungry for high-calorie protein, fat, and salt foods. This is precisely where pizza, Mexican, Italian, and fast food cravings come from. The end result is that you will need to overeat to finally get enough dopamine and leptin in the brain to shut down NPY and feel energized and focused once again. By then, the cost will have been too much – you'll have already overeaten, gained weight, and your blood sugar will have spiked.

Likewise, when leptin resistant diabetics have stress cravings for carbs and fat due to low serotonin, they will not be able to get enough leptin in the brain to shut down NPY before overeating on doughnuts, candy bars, or ice cream. Again, to finally feel relaxed and satisfied from eating, you'll have eaten too much. You're still hungry, irritable, and anxious despite eating – it solves nothing and makes you fatter with higher blood sugar. As the stress wears down your levels of serotonin and dopamine, you'll become a carb-or salty-fat-craving machine. This is where stress cravings come from.[15]

Another way that leptin increases appetite is by increasing ghrelin, a hormone in your stomach that gives you those hunger pangs, telling you to eat. Decreasing NPY also decreases ghrelin, but in diabetic or obese individuals, NPY and ghrelin are higher than normal. This means the physical and conscious desire to eat is higher and more frequent in diabetic and overweight people than non-diabetics. Ghrelin does not subside as quickly in diabetics and overweight people, which means they don't receive the signal to stop eating as soon. So NPY in the brain is not lowered as soon, which increases the duration of the meal and the likelihood to overeat. This is one reason why determining hours before what you are going to eat, and premeasuring that amount through an already prepared meal, will go a long way in preventing you from overeating when you're the most susceptible. So what's the solution?

> **For diabetics, the solution starts when you ditch the fast food dinner, acknowledge that you are under stress, and change your habits to better meet the increased demands on your time and energy.**

This may mean cutting back on those demands, but if you value the quality of your life, you'll do it.

We Control Diabetes to Control Its Complications

While diabetes is a disease with the symptoms of high blood sugar and obesity, you really want to see diabetes as a gateway disease.

> **It's not the excess glucose or pounds themselves that are going to get you. It's the consequences on the body as a result of having these two problems that explain why having diabetes is bad.**

Doctors attribute these consequences to vascular disease, referring to the blocking of blood flow from the largest arteries down to the smallest blood vessels. This one problem causes tremendous devastation.

The National Institutes of Health (NIH) has gathered the following statistics on diabetic vascular complications.[1]

- 68% of all diabetics die of heart disease and 16% from stroke. Diabetics have a two- to four-times greater chance of having a stroke or heart attack.
- Diabetes is the leading cause of blindness over age twenty and there are 18,000 new cases of diabetic eye disease each year.
- Diabetes is the leading cause of kidney failure, accounting for 44% of all new cases.
- About two-thirds of all diabetics have neuropathy.
- 60% of all nontraumatic amputations each year are performed on diabetics.

The gateway disease brought on by diabetes that causes these horrible consequences is called metabolic syndrome, which simply means having three or more of the following[20]:

- Abdominal obesity: A waist circumference of at least forty inches for men, and thirty-five inches for women (hence, the apple-shaped appearance).
- High triglycerides: 150 mg/dl or more.

- Low HDL cholesterol: Less than 40 mg/dl for men and 50 mg/dl for women.
- High blood pressure: At least 135/85 mm Hg. In fact, the NIH found 75% of all diabetics had blood pressure higher than 130/80 mm Hg.
- High fasting blood sugar: At least 110 mg/dl.

There are other ways to make vascular complications worse besides having metabolic disease or diabetes:

- Cigarette smoking: the more you smoke and the longer, the greater the risk. Smoking decreases the oxygen supply in the blood while increasing the heart's need for oxygen. This double whammy stresses the cardiovascular system. Do what you must to quit.
- Obesity: the more you weigh, the more stress on the body.
- Lack of exercise: exercise decreases blood pressure, cholesterol, glucose, and weight, so it's no wonder *lack* of exercise is a risk factor for heart attacks and strokes.

These account for all the risk factors that are within your control. Factors that increase the chance of getting a heart attack or stroke outside of your control include your age, sex (more likely in males), and family history of atherosclerosis, the hardening of the arteries.

It is still unclear whether metabolic disease is the cause or consequence of insulin resistance. What is clear is that if you're a diabetic, you probably have both. Most diabetics have a combination of high blood sugar coupled with high cholesterol, blood pressure, or triglycerides. All these issues came about from high insulin levels that went undetected for years, silently damaging your body by adding layer upon layer of fat, especially around your middle.

The take-home message is that all aspects of the metabolic syndrome are life threatening, not just the high blood sugar. As you now understand, very few people die from acutely high blood sugar. And while losing weight, exercising, and eating well can dramatically protect against all complications from diabetes, you need to have a firm grasp on what you're up against to know what you're fighting, and to motivate you to fight harder.

Macrovascular Disease: Heart Attacks, Strokes, and Peripheral Artery Disease

> **Nearly six out of seven diabetics will die from heart disease or stroke, and peripheral artery disease (PAD) will cause the greatest number of amputations each year[1].**

They are different diseases with the same cause – obstruction of blood flow through the arteries.

Diabetes increases the amount of low-density lipoproteins (LDLs) that deposits cholesterol along the inner lining of the arterial walls. It also decreases the amount of high-density lipoproteins (HDLs) that could have transported that junk all the way to the liver for disposal instead of dumping it in your arteries like trash on the freeway. This excess cholesterol, fat, and plaque then impact you in two major ways.

First, the formation of fat pads and blood clots along the arterial lining narrows and hardens the walls, stiffening them to cause ischemia, a restriction in blood supply. In the chest, this process can kill heart tissue, leading to a heart attack. If the ischemia happens closer to the brain, the result is a stroke. When it happens in the arms and legs, the lack of oxygen and blood flow coupled with neuropathy described below can cause infections from unfelt injuries to the feet, or even worse, gangrene, requiring amputation. Second, the stiffening of the arterial walls restricts blood flow, which increases blood pressure. And all of this happened from excess sludge just hanging out in your arteries.

In short, diabetes kills you slowly because it makes blood flow harder by giving you high blood pressure, cholesterol, and triglycerides. So it makes sense that you should care about controlling these factors as much as controlling your blood sugar.

Microvascular Disease: Blindness, Nerve Damage, and Kidney Failure

The obstruction of blood flow does not just occur in the big arteries. It can occur in the smaller blood vessels as well. You read how glycation damages the small blood vessels, allowing protein to leak out and blood flow to slow down. In the eyes, the excess fluid and protein builds up behind the retina, putting pressure on it that leads to blindness known as diabetic retinopathy.

In the kidneys, the damaged small blood vessels leak proteins that can strain the organs, leading to kidney disease known as diabetic nephropathy. Again, this is the leading cause of kidney disease.

As the lack of blood flow damages nerve cells, toes and feet become numb, and diabetic neuropathy occurs. Once you can no longer feel your feet stepping on a nail or being burned on hot ground, infection can set in that, if left unchecked, will require amputating a foot or toe to save your life.

Again, all this damage occurs from lack of blood flow. It should be clear to you now that we want to not only control blood sugar, but to directly do everything we can to ensure macrovascular and microvascular diseases never occur, or to diminish them if they already have.

The First Prescription: Be Accountable and Take Control

Your first prescription is to see where you stand with your health so *you* can take control of it. This will require you to get with your doctor about monitoring your medication dosage as you change your eating, exercise, and lifestyle – because you'll need his or her help to safely and gradually make the shift in diabetes treatment from meds first to meds last. This will require a shift in your relationship with your doctor, one that will likely be welcomed. I've never met a doctor who wasn't happy that a patient was taking his or her health seriously.

In his book *Taking Control of Your Diabetes*, Dr. Steven Edelman, himself a type I diabetic (see TCOYD.org), says that your doctor should check your weight, blood pressure, A1c, and feet every three to twelve months depending on severity[21]. At least once a year, your doctor should also check your fasting cholesterol, kidney health, thyroid, teeth, heart, and gastrointestinal system as needed. She may also test for neuropathy (peripheral nerve damage) and retinopathy (optic nerve damage).

Other measurements, such as your energy level and how much you sleep, are also very important. As you'll learn, quality sleep has a major impact on your blood sugar . For example, sleep apnea, an all-too-common disorder among overweight diabetics, makes glucose control and weight loss even harder. So you'll want to be honest with your doctor about all the symptoms you're experiencing.

You won't always have to schedule an appointment with your doctor to get these tests done, so that's no excuse. There are now fairly accurate home tests for your A1c and micro albumin levels, and your cholesterol can easily be checked at most drugstores.

You have to believe that you can change. You have to believe that no matter how much the scale has gone up in the past, it can start to trend down. You have to believe that no matter how high your morning readings have been, they can be lower. You have to believe that, and then you have to repeat the action that makes that happen over and over again.

Below are the desired ranges for all the blood and urine tests discussed thus far. Remember that whatever your numbers are at this point, these are just numbers, just starting points upon which to improve. That's all that matters. Whatever complications you're facing, and no matter how daunting they seem, there is no problem that cannot be made drastically better and maybe even solved.

The HbA1c: The Diabetic Complication Yardstick

The first number you absolutely must know is your percentage of glycated hemoglobin, or HbA1c. Every diabetic should be familiar with this blood test and term: it's your three-month average blood sugar reading. In simple terms, it measures how much sugar is "sticking to your blood," how glycated your blood cells have become. The more glycated your blood cells, the higher your blood sugar's been.

A glycation of 6% is considered the high end of normal, and correlates to an average blood sugar of 120 mg/dl. As a diabetic, your ultimate goal is to have an A1c of less than 7.0%, corresponding to an average glucose reading of less than 150 mg/dl. That's the blood sugar level that the 1993 Diabetes Control and Complications Trial (DCCT), a nine-year, 1,400-person, $160-million study, and the most extensive longitudinal study ever done on diabetes, found to be at the lowest risk for complications[22]. The DCCT was aimed at type I diabetics, and a follow-up study on type II diabetics, known as the United Kingdom Prospective Diabetes Study (UKPDS), validated the same conclusion for the type II's[23].

> **These studies proved to the medical community that tight glucose control could delay, if not altogether stop, the progression of complications from diabetes.**

An A1c of 7.0% or lower was shown to have a lot of advantages:

- Blood sugar control reduced the chance of developing new retinopathy by 76% in those studied, and delayed progression in those who already had eye disease by 54%.
- There was a statistically significant decrease in nerve and kidney disease compared to the control group.
- Patients in the tight glucose control group reported a

higher quality of life, and did not feel that the rigors of tight control adversely affected their lives. They reported a decrease in excessive thirst, daytime tiredness, poor wound healing, and blurry vision.

In contrast, every increase of 1% in A1c over 8.0% also increased the risk of eye disease from 40 to 50%. That equates to a three-month average blood sugar reading of 180 mg/dl or higher. A 1.0% increase in A1c equates to having an average blood sugar that is 30mg/dl higher, so going from an average blood sugar of 180 mg/dl to 210 mg/dl or higher is devastating as far as your body is concerned. On the good side, lowering the A1c will very likely mean that your blood pressure and cholesterol are well under control.

The only downfall here is that the A1c rating is an average. If you spend half the time at 50 mg/dl, and the other half at 250 mg/dl, that's an average of 150 mg/dl, an HbA1c of around 7%. However, without taking insulin, such spreads between highs and lows are less likely.

Below 6.0% is ideal, but below 7.0% is acceptable. You should have this checked every three months or as often as your doctor says. There are even home kits you can buy at your local pharmacist if you want to save the trip to the doctor's office.

Test Your Blood Sugar Daily[21]

While the A1c is a great tool for you and your doctor to check the severity of your diabetes, you do need to check your blood sugar daily at specific times.

Fasting Blood Sugar: Your blood sugar when you wake up before you eat or drink anything. Less than 100 mg/dl is ideal, but less than 120 mg/dl is acceptable.

PostPrandial Blood Sugar: Your blood sugar sixty to ninety minutes after finishing your meal. Less than 120 mg/dl one to two hours after eating is ideal, but 140 to 180 mg/dl in that time frame is acceptable.

PrePrandial Blood Sugar: Your blood sugar before you eat. Less than 115 mg/dl is ideal, but less than 120 mg/dl is acceptable.

Bedtime Blood Sugar: Your blood sugar before you go to bed. Less than 120 mg/dl is ideal, 140 mg/dl is acceptable, but a minimum of 100 mg/dl is desirable when using insulin or any insulin secretagogue capable of causing nighttime hypoglycemia.

Hypoglycemia: When you're on prescription drugs to treat diabetes, your blood sugar can sometimes dip too low. If this happens recurrently for years, you can even develop a degree of hypoglycemic unawareness, where you no longer feel the sudden onset of shaking, rapid heartbeat, and sweating to alert you to the problem.

Be on the lookout if your blood sugar dips below 70 mg/dl. If it does, drink some fruit juice or have some glucose tablets, roughly 10 to 20 grams of sugar. Then retest. Have no fat or protein in the meal so blood sugar may rise as quickly as possible, the exact opposite of what you normally want. You are treating a potentially life-threatening condition, not going for fine cuisine. Your doctor or pharmacist should have already instructed you on what to look out for and what to do.

Prescription Glucose Strips: You can often get the most state-of-the-art glucometers for free because the drug companies make their money by overcharging you for the glucose strips that come with the meter. You see, only particular glucose strips work for a particular meter, and a box of strips can cost over $70 without a prescription. But you can drastically lessen the cost of glucose strips by first always having your doctor prescribe them to you instead of buying them over the counter, and second, always having your doctor prescribe 200 strips at a time. A box of glucose strips usually has 100 strips, but if your doctor prescribes you two boxes at a time (i.e., 200 strips), you'll still have the same copay as a one-box prescription. At $70 per box of 100 strips, and $20 per copay for two boxes, these two tricks reduce the cost per strip from 70 cents to 10 cents. This is the only prescription I now have for my diabetes.

The Tape Measurer and Scale: How to Track Weight Loss Progress

Since losing weight is the most natural "cure" for type II diabetes, you'll need to weigh yourself weekly, in the morning, after having gone to the bathroom, and before eating or drinking anything. You should also check your fat loss with measurements every week in the following five areas: waist, hips, chest, upper arms, and upper thigh. Add these numbers together, and watch the sum reduce month by month. You'll likely see the waist measurement drop the most over time as that is where diabetics store most of their fat. No one needs to know these numbers but you. It doesn't even matter what they are. It only matters whether they're going up or down over time. Losing weight will make more of a difference in every facet of diabetes than anything else you could do.

Measuring body fat loss with a tape measure is easy, but it will not indicate your body fat percentage. Ideally, you want your body fat to be below 20% if male, and 30% if female. These are both the high end of normal body fat, indicating you are not overweight below these values.

A body mass index (BMI) is the tool your doctor will invariably use to measure your body fat. It's a way to compare how much weight you carry relative to your height.

$$\text{BMI} = \text{Weight (lb)} \times 703 \div \text{Height}^2 \text{ (in}^2\text{)}$$

A BMI from 18.5 to 25 is considered normal, 25 to 30 is overweight, 30 to 35 is stage I obese, 35 to 40 stage II obese, and 40 or more is stage III obese. The formula can be very misleading in weight lifters who carry a lot of muscle. However, if you carry too much fat and lead a sedentary lifestyle, this formula will probably be accurate in measuring how overweight you are. For example, at my heaviest of 220 pounds and 65.5 inches, my BMI was hovering around 36, which put me at Stage II Obese. Today, at 155 pounds, my BMI is 25, the high end of what's considered normal weight, but my body fat is low. Lifting weights has now thrown my BMI off in terms of measuring how fat I am. Back then, it was spot on.

Besides getting your total body fat down, you also want to get your waist measurement to drop as quickly as possible, as visceral fat is an independent marker for heart disease and stroke. Men should have a waist measurement lower than forty inches, and women less than thirty-five inches.

Cholesterol and Blood Pressure Must Be Checked and Controlled[21]

High cholesterol and high blood pressure are both known as silent killers because they have no symptoms for a long time. It's important to identify these problems early so you can live a long healthy life. Besides going to your doctor, you can also get a lipid profile at most pharmacies.

Blood Pressure: A reading of 120/80 mm Hg is ideal, but a reading of 130/80 mm Hg is acceptable.

Triglycerides: This is a measurement of fat in the blood. Less than 150 mg/dl is ideal if you've already suffered a heart attack, stroke, or congestive heart failure, but less than 200 mg/dl is acceptable if you have not.

Low-Density Lipoprotein (LDL): This is the bad cholesterol that clogs the arteries. Less than 70 mg/dl is ideal if you've already suffered a heart attack, stroke, or congestive heart failure, but less than 100 mg/dl is acceptable if you have not.

High-Density Lipoprotein (HDL): This is the good one because it clears the bad cholesterol from the blood vessels. Greater than 50 mg/dl for women and 40 mg/dl for men is ideal.

Total Cholesterol: This is the sum of HDL and LDL. Less than 200 mg/dl is ideal, but you should make sure such a reading isn't because your HDL is too low and your LDL too high – that will still put you at extreme risk for a heart attack.

Monitor the Health of Your Kidneys[21]

Micro albumin: A reading of 30 to 300 mg/dl is a sign of kidney damage (though healthy kidney function usually means zero micro albumin in the urine).

Albumin-to-Creatinine Ratio: More than 2.8 g/mmol if male and 2.0 mg/mmol if female are both signs of nephropathy.

Get Your Eyes, Feet, and Thyroid Checked[21]

Eyes: Your doctor will refer you to a specialist at regular intervals to test for diabetic retinopathy. Depending on the state of your eyes, treatments will vary.

Feet: Your doctor will refer you to a specialist at regular intervals to test for diabetic neuropathy. Depending on the state of your feet and nerves, treatments will vary.

TSH (thyroid-stimulating hormone): TSH tests whether your metabolism is sluggish due to a suboptimally functioning thyroid. A reading of 0.4-2.5 uIU/mL is healthy in most adults.

With these measurements in hand, you and your doctor can now do the most important thing with them – check them again and again, and seek to improve them over time. That is the point, right? The idea is to improve these values, no matter how abysmal they may be initially, right? They're not meant to be ignored. They're not meant to be given due consideration for a week, but then fall out of conscious thought beneath more meaningful numbers like taxes, gas prices, and credit card bills. They're not there just so doctors can pretend to have done something, or to give you the impression that lowering them is someone else's responsibility. Rather, the idea behind these tests is to give you power, the power of knowing where you are, and where you need to be.

What I Want You to Check

I want you to keep track of the following each and every day. This is so you can start changing some of the behaviors that have made your diabetes occur in the first place. Whether or not

Be Accountable and Take Control

WHAT'S TESTED	WHY TESTED	HOW MEASURED	WHO MEASURES	HOW OFTEN	IDEAL TARGET
Blood Sugar	Glycation causes every problem below	Blood test and glucometer	You with glucometer and your doctor with A1c	Every day with glucometer and every 3 months with A1c	Under 100 mg/dl fasting, 120 mg/dl after meals, 6.0% A1c
Blood Pressure	Causes heart attacks and strokes, killing 6 out of 7 diabetics	Blood pressure cuff	You at home and your doctor at checkups	Every day or as recommended by doctor	Less than 120/80 mm Hg
Blood Cholesterol	Causes heart attacks and strokes, killing 6 out of 7 diabetics	Blood test	Your doctor or pharmacist	Every 3 months or as recommended by doctor	Under 150 mg/dl triglycerides, 70 mg/dl LDL, and over 50 mg/dl HDL (40 if female)
Weight & Body Fat	Weight loss is unanimously by far the best and only cure for type II diabetes	Scale and tape measurer	You do	Once a week in morning after bathroom	BMI under 25 and body fat less than 20% (30% if female)
Kidneys	Diabetes is the leading cause of kidney disease	Blood & urine test	Your doctor at checkups	Every 6 months or as recommended by doctor	No protein at all in urine, and less than 2.8 g/mmol albumin-to-creatinine ratio (2.0 if female)
Eyes	Diabetes is the leading cause of adult blindness	Medical exam	Your doctor or specialist	Every 6 months or as recommended by doctor	Consult your physician for what's right for you. Ideally, no retinopathy
Feet	Diabetes is the leading cause of neuropathy	Medical exam	Your doctor or specialist	Every 6 months or as recommended by doctor	Consult your physician for what's right for you. Ideally, no neuropathy
Thyroid	Indicates metabolism is slow, making weight loss harder	Blood test	Your doctor at checkups	Every 6 months or as recommended by doctor	TSH reading of 0.4-2.5 uIU/mL

diabetes runs in our families, it was our behaviors that made it possible. Whether or not there was dynamite in our house, we were the ones who lit the match. For that reason, track the following.

- How many sodas you drink per day.
- How much fast food you eat every day.
- How much other junk food you eat every day.
- How often after consuming the items above you eat again, and what.
- How much exercise you do per day.

And Now Let's Cut To The Chase...

I spent the first part of this chapter outlining how diabetes got to be so bad. Thing is, I'll bet you'd already made the connection between obesity, overeating, and diabetes in your mind. You knew those doughnut breakfasts, candy bar lunches, and fast food dinners (I know I'm not the only one) were a problem just as much as I did when I was first diagnosed.

> I'll bet you also knew exercising, eating better, and losing weight would make a profound difference in your blood sugar, cholesterol, and blood pressure. So I have to ask...*why haven't you changed already?*

Since controlling diabetes is a day-to-day process, let me make the question simpler by asking you some questions about your day-to-day life.

One: What is it about controlling your diabetes that would feel better than any food could ever taste?

Two: Why would it be worth it to you to prepare meals or exercise even if it meant skipping TV?

Three: What would motivate you to exercise no matter how tired or busy or stressed you were?

Four: What would motivate you to skip the bread, eat half the dessert, and not ask for seconds?

Do you see the theme? I'm really asking for your reasons to lose weight, exercise, eat better, and do it again the next day. What feels better than chocolate could ever taste? What could make you think twice about the dessert table again, and again, and again?

If you can't come up with the answer, you'll never make it.

I'll give you mine. I love the feeling of being awake, alert, and alive. I hate feeling tired and bloated after eating poorly. So I love foods that make me lean and awake. It actually makes me not like dessert unless I know it will help me become leaner (which it can as you'll learn).

To take that one step further, I know that my life is meant to help people, and I know that I can't do that if I'm tired or don't feel good about myself. So eating and exercising in this way are directly in line with my life mission. My reasons are entirely authentic to me, so when I'm faced with the dessert table, my set motivations are sweeter than the foods in front of me, enough to pull me away from what could destroy me.

| **What I'm asking you is very simple: who are you?**

So this is who I am. What I'm asking you is very simple: who are you? Put the book down until you know.

Now That You Know, You Can Heal

You now understand why diabetes is so deadly, what its complications are, and how they're measured. You know what causes diabetes, and you now know why you want to heal. However, I'm not going to tell you to go on a low-carb diet and start exercising just yet. First, we have to deal with what really got you to become 50, 150, or 250 pounds overweight. I know my own answer because I've been there myself.

What drove you to sit on your butt, stuff your gut, and get in a rut? Diabetes is really a disease of excessive cravings, fat storage, and vascular problems. If you treat the desire to overeat the wrong foods, you'll lose the weight and directly attack the vascular disease. *Then,* **you'll be controlling diabetes. So we must first attack the need to eat junk. In other words,** *we need to deal with our emotional eating...*

The First Prescription in Summary

- There is no pill that can "cure" diabetes and make you lose all the weight.
- One in three Americans born after 2000 will get diabetes, the fastest rate ever in the history of the human race. Our genes have not changed in the past 10,000 years. Our lifestyle and food has.
- High blood sugar is the number one symptom of type II diabetes. Insulin resistance is the cause.
- In turn, insulin resistance is caused by overeating, inactivity, and weight gain.
- In turn, these three factors bring on insulin resistance via excess sugar, insulin, and fat in the blood.
- Stress makes diabetes worse by causing excess cortisone and adrenaline resistance, both making fat loss harder. Eating a diet high in sugar and processed carbs makes it even worse.
- Leptin is the hormone that travels from your fat cells to your brain so the hypothalamus can regulate your appetite and metabolic rate.
- The same problems that cause insulin resistance in the body lead to leptin resistance in the brain. The result is greater cravings for carbohydrates and decreased metabolism, making diabetes and weight

gain even harder to reverse.

- Diabetes is such a serious condition because it causes vascular disease, the blockage of blood flow through the body. It comes in two flavors – macrovascular and microvascular disease.
- Macrovascular disease in diabetics is responsible for heart attacks, strokes, and peripheral artery disease.
- Microvascular disease in diabetics is responsible for kidney disease, eye disease, and neuropathy.
- The First Prescription is all about taking control of your own health. That means knowing where you stand with your diabetes and complications.
- Your first goal is to get your HbA1c down to at least below 7.0%, the lower the better.
- You will measure your weight loss using a scale and tape measure weekly.
- You also want to know where you stand with your blood pressure, cholesterol, thyroid, kidneys, eyes, and feet. Your doctor will check all of these for you.
- You will never recover from diabetes unless you can answer why it's really worth it to you to change.

"We earn diabetes through our actions, admittedly helped by a family history."

2

SECOND PRESCRIPTION

Control Emotional Eating to Control Blood Sugar

*W*elcome to my hell. *There's talk and laughter all around, but all I can think about is what I'm about to eat. I'm sitting at the table, scanning the menu thoroughly. What's the biggest thing I can find? It has to taste good. I'm so anxious that I can't stop fidgeting under the table. I have this knot just below my heart that won't go away. I hope my girlfriend doesn't notice. After dinner, I want a tiramisu. I hope I don't have to share. The only thing I don't like about tiramisu is that it's so small. I wish this place had banana splits. The gnocchi looks good…oh great, here's the bread. This place has the best olive oil dip for their bread…*

I can't believe I finished my gnocchi so fast. I'm not hungry, but I want to keep eating. At least there's still bread. Won't everyone just hurry up and finish so we can order dessert? Hendry is going on about the strife in Peru. He's so passionate about the problems of his country. But I can't stop staring at his plate of linguini. He's just holding his fork, forgetting to eat as he goes on and on. How can he do that? He just came off a six-hour shift at the homeless shelter, and he's not eating? How the hell does he do that? Oh good, Alex is full from his ravioli. I can have the rest of his plate. This will at least hold me until Hendry finishes his dinner and we can order dessert. I really need to stop doing this. I know I'm full, but it's never enough. Tonight is blown anyways, and I am having dessert. After all, it's my birthday...

— My thoughts on the weekend of my twenty-second birthday
Steps of Rome restaurant, San Francisco, California

Emotional Eating Is the Spark That Lit the Dynamite

Food is the most commonly abused drug on the planet. Almost everyone living in a First or Second World country has at one time or another used food to soothe themselves, numb their feelings, or relieve boredom. We've all overeaten from time to time. We go out for a big dinner, have a dessert with coffee, and leave uncomfortably stuffed. But that doesn't mean you have a problem with overeating. Just as almost everyone has had an alcoholic drink, not everyone is an alcoholic.

But there are those of us for whom emotional eating is a very big problem. Most diabetics have accelerated the progression of their disease through overeating. We didn't get this disease by eating celery and hard-boiled eggs; we weren't skinny around the middle when we got this disease; we hadn't just completed training for a marathon when we got this disease. Diabetes is a disease of a sedentary lifestyle as much as it is one of overeating junk food. The two go hand and hand.

> **This disease doesn't just "happen" to anyone
> – we earn diabetes through our actions,
> admittedly helped by a family history.**

It's not even enough to overeat and get fat to get diabetes. We type II's certainly aren't the only people in America to have gone on a candy raid. We're not the only ones who grab a Frappuccino and croissant in the morning without considering the consequences. We're not the only ones who stand by the dessert table and pick at it all night. We're not the only ones who order a large banana split after we've just finished a five-course meal or make midnight doughnut runs. Millions of Americans have the same addictions, but don't get diabetes. What's the difference between us and them?

You have to have the genes for diabetes to get diabetes – if you just live a sedentary lifestyle and overeat junk food without that genetic predisposition, you'll just wind up overweight but not diabetic. But even if you have that genetic predisposition, you probably can't get diabetes unless you express it through your behavior. The behavior is not exercising while overeating junk food to satisfy the body's cravings. That's why emotional eating is so dangerous for diabetics.

> **The potential to get sick was there at birth, but overeating is the vehicle that gets you there.**

After we're diagnosed, all of us go through some sort of check list of past activities we may have done to exacerbate our condition. One diabetic man told me his Friday night ritual used to be an entire bucket of extra crispy fried chicken with a gallon of mint chip ice cream; another diabetic woman told me she used to eat chocolate cake every day. Why is it so hard for alcoholics to recover? Because they love to drink. Why is it so hard for diabetics to recover? Because we love our food. Whether we emotionally eat more than non-diabetics or just suffer more, either way, we need to stop. Just because everyone else is doing it does not make it OK.

Emotional Eating Is Defined through Its Excessiveness

Emotional eating, which I'll lump together with binge eating and overeating, is defined as eating excessive amounts of food for any reason other than to meet your nutritional requirements. That definition does *not* imply that you shouldn't enjoy eating. If you enjoy your meal while fueling your body without overeating, then you have *not* emotionally eaten. However, if you overeat, regardless of how nutritious the meal, then you *have* emotionally eaten. The snapshot from my past described above gives a perfect example of emotional eating – I didn't need all that food – I just wanted it. Why I wanted all that food is not necessary to call it emotional eating. The fact that I didn't need to consume 3,000 calories at dinner to satisfy my body's energy requirements, but I did anyway, pretty much seals the deal. Further, the reasons behind emotional eating often have less to do with what's going on inside your *mind*, and more to do with what's going on inside your *brain*. As you'll learn in this section, your brain and body usually influence your mind to want to eat more. It's usually not the other way around.

Defining emotional eating as we have begs the question, how do you know when you've eaten too much? Logically, we can compare how many calories you've eaten to how many calories you've burned today, plus consider your food's nutritional quality.

> **Practically, it comes down to common sense. There's eating a bowl of ice cream, and then there's eating a gallon of ice cream. There's eating ice cream once in a while, and then there's eating ice cream every day.**

Even worse, there's eating a gallon of ice cream every day. Just as occasionally drinking doesn't make you an alcoholic, occasionally eating junk food doesn't make you an emotional eater. However, eating a lot of junk food a lot of the time probably does. And if you're diabetic, that emotional eating is your worst enemy. Exercise can't stop the fat gained from binging on 3,500 calories worth of cookies and pizza once or twice a week. The excess calories, wrought with refined carbs and saturated fats, make losing weight and controlling blood sugar impossible.

Therefore, you must master the solutions below to control emotional eating to control diabetes.

As I've previously alluded to, emotional eating is also hard to define because the very term is a misnomer. "Emotional" eating suggests people overeat to satisfy an emotional void. That is not entirely accurate. We now know there are numerous physiological processes that influence our desire for different foods. Some people are more genetically predisposed to overeat; what we eat influences what we'll be tempted to eat next; whether we're overweight, whether we're well rested, whether we're stressed, whether we've exercised, and of course our emotions all influence our cravings.

> **Diabetics beware, because due to our abnormally high and low swinging blood sugars, just being a type II diabetic has also been shown not only to lock in the pattern of craving certain foods, but also causes us to not feel full or satisfied on a "normal" sized meal.**

My aim then in this section is to educate you on the factors that influence us to want to eat foods high in sugar and fat and how to *not* have these cravings anymore. The craving for something rich and sugary has great significance to your brain, and understanding that significance will go a long way toward helping you avoid emotionally eating so you can lose weight to control diabetes and its complications.

- Emotional eating is any eating done in excess that does not meet your body's nutritional requirements. It has nothing to do with whether or not you enjoy the meal.
- Emotional eating is more of an imbalance in your brain chemistry than in your feelings.
- The most common craving is for sugar and fat together, such as in doughnuts, chocolate, ice cream, and cheesecake.

Knowing Why You're Craving Sugar and Fat Is the Key to Solving Your Emotional Eating

> We never crave foods haphazardly – every craving
> serves a need to the mind, brain, and body.

Biologically, emotional eating boils down to the functionality of neurotransmitters like serotonin, GABA, and dopamine, and hormones like insulin, leptin, and cortisone. These are the brain chemicals that influence appetite, cravings, and pleasure. Like your friends, they tempt you with fried chicken and ice cream, share in the joy of eating it, and console you afterward when you're feeling guilty about indulging in them. Like your enemies, when they work against you, they don't help you fall off the wagon – they pick you up and throw you off. The interplay between these brain chemicals sets you up to crave more and more of the same damaging foods once you start eating them, locking in the habit of craving the wrong foods in the wrong amounts. This chapter will teach you what contributes to sugar and fat cravings and how to stop them. Every craving has a chemical.

Why You Get Those Cookie, Candy, and Ice Cream Cravings

Cravings for sugar and fat are created by your brain to raise serotonin, a major neurotransmitter. Examples of sugar and fat cravings would be chocolate, ice cream, cake, cookies, and pancakes with butter. By understanding your brain's purposes behind giving you this craving, you can understand how to effectively shut it off without resorting to 1,000-calorie binges.

Serotonin's influence on appetite is at least partially due to how its receptors in the brain work.[22] If serotonin is a baseball, its receptor in the brain is the catcher. As a neurotransmitter, serotonin plays many roles in the brain, stabilizing mood, managing pain, and even regulating blood pressure. Its receptors have even been shown to improve glucose tolerance.[23] Selective serotonin reuptake inhibitors (SSRIs) like Prozac, prescribed for clinical depression, increase the brain's supply of serotonin. SSRIs are generally prescribed to help take the "edge" off of depression by causing more serotonin to remain active in the brain. However, Prozac is also prescribed sometimes for emotional eating because serotonin induces satiety and alleviates food cravings, specifically those for carbohydrates. When serotonin levels in the brain are low, they stimulate the body's appetite control centers, causing a craving for high-carbohydrate foods.[1]

Why carbohydrates? The answer is very simple: consuming carbohydrates increases serotonin levels. The body builds serotonin from the amino acid tryptophan, a protein component found in every piece of cheese, milk, and egg you've ever eaten. Meanwhile sugar, the simplest carbohydrate, triggers the body to increase the amount of serotonin in the brain.[1] In layman's terms, carbohydrates (sugar) cause the body to release feel-good chemicals. Eating a doughnut leads to a complex chemical process that makes you actually feel calmer and happier.

It's important to understand that while carbohydrates increase total serotonin, serotonin is first built from tryptophan. A low-protein diet means that the body can't make enough serotonin due to a lack of tryptophan. Because serotonin will be lower, you will subconsciously crave carbohydrates because the brain and body know that carbs can boost serotonin. This process was proven in the lab when two researchers at MIT fed a group of people and animals a diet intentionally low in the amino acid tryptophan—*all of them* became hungrier for carbohydrates.[2] They didn't want protein even though that's where serotonin comes from – they wanted carbs, not protein, when they were restricted from eating protein. The lesson then is clear.

> **A cornerstone to controlling emotional eating is to make sure you're having a serving of protein at *every* meal.**

As the above experiment shows, eating protein can reduce your cravings for carbohydrates. Besides cravings for cookies and milk, other symptoms of low serotonin include headaches, insomnia, fatigue, moodiness, depression, anxiety, and increased hunger at night. Does this sound a little like PMS? It should, because many of the symptoms of PMS are correlated with the decreased serotonin levels that occur prior to menstruation.[3] But women *and* men need to care about serotonin because the symptoms should also sound familiar to diabetics. For the entire population, the substances we consume day to day affect how much, or how little, serotonin is floating around in our brain. You're building your near future appetite at this very moment.

What you eat or drink now affects what you'll want to eat or drink a few hours from now.

Low serotonin is the reason why anyone who is depressed or nervous, or anyone running on four hours of sleep, reaches for high-sugar and high-fat foods like cookies, candy, and ice cream. Fat, like carbohydrates, helps boost serotonin levels. For diabetics, since we already have a chemical imbalance in our blood, this bodily awareness of serotonin is far greater than in the general population. We must be even more careful of what we eat and how it affects us, both physically and emotionally. One alcoholic drink affects someone with a liver disorder far worse than anyone of average health. Likewise, one binge affects a diabetic far worse than a non-diabetic. We're more affected through our propensity to gain fat and experience high blood sugar. Now that we know low serotonin causes carbohydrate and fat cravings, we need to understand how serotonin gets low in the first place.

- Low serotonin in the brain causes cravings for sugar and fat together, such as in cereal, candy, chocolate, ice cream, doughnuts, cookies, cakes, and pastries.
- Serotonin is built from the amino acid tryptophan,

but amplified through sugar and fat; a low-protein diet will cause carbohydrate cravings for this reason.

- Besides cravings for carbohydrates, other symptoms of low serotonin include headaches, insomnia, fatigue, moodiness, depression, anxiety, and increased hunger at night; the symptoms mirror those of PMS.
- Diabetics are even more susceptible to emotional eating from their swinging insulin levels.[7]

Serotonin Drops From Physical and Mental Stress

A drop in serotonin doesn't happen on its own. Neither do the cravings that come with that drop. The whole process usually starts when internal or external stressors overwhelm your body, which causes serotonin levels to drop, triggering the desire for sugar and fat to replenish serotonin in the brain.[4] Those stressors come from a combination of three factors – your genes, behaviors, and cognitions, a.k.a. your thoughts and feelings. Every stress you experienced that ended in you staring down the bottom of a gallon of ice cream could be explained from a combination of those three factors. In this case, stress doesn't necessarily mean too much work; it's anything that overwhelms the body's operating system. Further, not all people handle the same stress the same. If you and I are both diabetics who eat two pieces of cake after performing the exact same stressful tasks, my cravings for more cake might be five times the strength of yours due to different genes.

But how genetic is emotional eating? It's different for everyone. You can be predisposed at birth to feel less satisfied from food, causing you to want to eat more than normal; you can be predisposed to swinging blood sugar that causes cravings when you crash; you can be a more anxious, depressed person naturally due to lower serotonin or other neurotransmitters.

> **Still, there is no gene that specifically makes you want ice cream. But no matter what hand was dealt you through your genes, you don't have to accept it as your fate.**

If scientists find that you have a genetic propensity to want to shoot yourself in the head, does that make it OK? Just as with anything else, we ultimately get to choose how we live our lives. In the end, it's neither our genes, nor our bodies, nor our brains, but our minds that chose what goes in our mouths. Your genes and behavior may push your cravings to the brink, but it's ultimately you who decides whether to pull the trigger.

> **There are countless behaviors we learn throughout our lifetime that teach us to treat food as a coping mechanism, emotional crutch, or mask for what we're going through emotionally.**

Everyone you know probably has a specific food they turn to as their "comfort food." Living in a First World country makes this even more likely. With an abundance of cheap, highly refined, high-calorie foods with little nutritional value, we Americans can prescribe ourselves as much food as we want to mask our emotional pain.

The strategy behind solving emotional eating is making the desire to eat well as easy as possible — we don't want emotional eating to even cross our minds. Unfortunately, we can't do much about our genes, and unraveling years of learned behaviors over a lifetime takes time. Therefore, we must battle our foe in the realm of our actions and behaviors. Fortunately for the sake of this strategy, our behaviors influence our serotonin levels the most by far.

The Behaviors That Feed the Cravings

If you're abusing alcohol, sweets, starches, or stimulants, cravings are inevitable. Low serotonin coupled with a diabetic's naturally swinging blood sugar is why you get hungry again two hours after having a high-sugar caffeinated beverage like soda or a mocha latte. Like sugar, caffeine causes a spike in insulin levels, which results in a blood sugar drop ninety minutes after consumption. In this case, we have two forces working to push blood sugar up and then down – you're going to get cravings! And blood sugar is irrevocably connected to serotonin: whenever blood sugar drops, serotonin falls as well. As we've seen, this causes carbohydrate cravings, which will fix the problem for about ninety minutes. Then blood sugar and serotonin levels crash again. It's a never-ending process. This means diabetics are especially prone to sugar and fat cravings from their behaviors.

Alcohol causes cravings because it lowers blood sugar by halting the creation of liver glycogen, a storage space for glucose. With the body's supply of glucose running low, your brain will lower its serotonin level to influence you to find something sweet – the fastest way to bring blood sugar back up. If you ever find yourself hungry an hour after having an alcoholic drink, you've just identified a behavior that adds to your emotional eating. ·

Stress can also cause severe cravings for carbohydrates. When stressed, adrenaline and cortisol work double duty to break down fats, proteins, and carbohydrates in the body to provide energy for the work at hand. But if stress becomes chronic, as it often can in our overworked world, your levels of cortisol and adrenaline can become inadequate, unable to meet your energy needs. All of a sudden, your body has become like a bank whose customers are all withdrawing their money at the same time. The body can't keep up with the demand, so it borrows energy once you feel worn out and have low blood sugar by influencing you to consume high-calorie foods.

Cortisol can also cause leptin and serotonin levels to drop,[4,5] a surefire way to slow metabolism and boost hunger. Lack of sleep, falling in love, losing your job, and a strong cup of coffee are all stresses that lead to the body releasing cortisol. This is yet another process that causes carb cravings. But sugar cravings aren't the only craving created by stress. Too little sleep and too much work can actually cause the cravings for nicotine, sugar, caffeine, or alcohol in the first place. If the brain and body can't adapt to whatever stress you're experiencing, they'll influence your behavior to help them out. In other words, emotional eating can come from the *body's* stress, just as much as from your own emotional stress over the day's occurrences.

Artificially sweetened products and diet soft drinks can also cause cravings[27]. Aspartame, saccharine, and Splenda are all hundreds of times sweeter than natural sugar and nearly calorie free. Scientists at Purdue University have noticed animals fed large amounts of artificial sweeteners stop associating the taste of sweet as being high in calories, leading to overconsumption of real and fake sugar foods. The last thing you want to do when trying to kill sugar cravings is to replace real sugar with fake sugar. As the study showed, that's only going to perpetuate the desire, not end it.

All five taste buds – bitter, sweet, sour, salty, and savory (think protein and fatty foods like steak) – can be overstimulated. If you eat only five grams of sugar a day, for example, a Popsicle with ten grams of sugar will taste very sweet.

> **However, if you regularly consume more than 100 grams of sugar every day, or even the "sweet" equivalent in artificial sweeteners from diet sodas and yellow, pink, and blue packets, you'll become accustomed to sugar and resistant to its effect, just as though it was a drug. You'll be able to eat 50 grams of it and still feel unsatisfied.**

You'll want and need more sugar, and your body will find a way to act on that need. Likewise, if you eat a lot of salt, your salt taste buds will become overstimulated, and you'll spend your time craving salt. The same goes for bitter, sour, and savory foods, although people tend to be more drawn to salty and sweet foods than the other three. Last and certainly not least, insulin resistance can literally tempt you to eat three times your daily food intake at one sitting. Too much insulin floating around the bloodstream will create a rapid drop in blood sugar, causing severe carbohydrate cravings, and opening the door for a major binge. The solution is to not eat high-carb, poor-quality foods that require a lot of insulin to process! The less insulin needed by the body, the less chance that your blood sugar will swing out of control and cause more cravings.

| **What you choose to eat creates your future appetite.** |

Reading all of this, you may think that cravings are our downfall. That's not true – it's how we usually deal with those cravings that is our diabetic downfall. Who says we can't find healthier ways to deal with them? The truth is we can. The take-home lesson is that since emotionally eating is founded both in the mind and the body, you have to attack it from both directions. What you eat sets you up to crave more and more of the right *or wrong* foods. It works both ways. The wrong carbs are addicting, and eating high fat and sugar snacks sets you up for more cravings. The next section will show you why, so you'll then be ready to learn how to appease cravings without gaining one pound of fat and two of guilt.

- Emotional eating is undeniably a learned behavior, but your genetic makeup, hormones, and neurotransmitters influence how "well" you learn it.[1] *It's not all just in your head.*
- Emotional eating must be dealt with biologically and psychologically. Ignore either and even the best nutritional and exercise program will not help you.
- Your behaviors influence your serotonin levels the most – caffeine, sugar, stress, little sleep, nicotine, dieting, alcohol, and swinging insulin levels all lower serotonin and induce carb cravings.

- Artificial sweeteners do not appease sugar cravings – they create sweet cravings. Abstaining from the taste of sugar kills sweet cravings.
- When you understand how what you eat sets you up for what you want to eat next, you'll be well on your way to ridding yourself of emotional eating forever, and making stable blood sugar and sustained fat loss a really possibility.
- Unfortunately, any boost in mood from gorging on sweets is only temporary. In the same way that a candy bar brings your blood sugar up and then causes a crash, that candy bar brings your serotonin level and mood up, and then back down.[6]

High Carb and High Calorie Are the Real Problem with This Craving

If you still don't think of high-carb foods as addictive, prepare yourself for an eye opener. "Our evidence … suggests that binge-ing on sugar can act in the brain in ways very similar to drugs of abuse," noted lead researcher Bart Hoebel, a professor of psychology at Princeton University, in a discussion with Amanda Gardner of *HealthDay*.[9] He went on to say that:

"Drinking large amounts of sugar water when hungry can cause behavioral changes and severe neurochemical changes in the brain which resemble changes that are produced when animals or people take substances of abuse. These animals show signs of withdrawal and even long-lasting effects that might resemble craving."

Sugar and enriched flour *can* be as addicting as cocaine.

This is why cutting out your harmful ways of eating is so hard even though you know you should. Three types of carbs that will prevail in your cravings and more than 99% of all emotional eating are white sugar, high-fructose corn syrup, and enriched (a.k.a. refined, bleached, or white) flour. Any of these three can be the main carbohydrate in sugar and fat craving. I single them out because their highly processed design gives your appetite no off switch and promotes fat gain, making them the most fattening calories in existence.

High-fructose corn syrup does not raise leptin, the metabolic master hormone that controls your metabolic rate and appetite.

> **By not raising leptin after a meal, high-fructose corn syrup goes unnoticed by your body's internal caloric accountants. Your brain basically thinks you didn't eat, so appetite remains high, forcing you to keep eating until you're satisfied. This break in your appetite feedback loop is why so many Americans can guzzle a two-liter bottle of soda and still be hungry even though the soda provided more than half the calories they need in a day.**

This is why you can go to your favorite fast food restaurant, down a large cheeseburger with fries, order a large soda, down it, refill it, down it again, and be hungry three hours later! Your body misread the 2,000 calories of sugar in the soda! **That's not supposed to happen!** Try that same trick with a calorically equivalent amount of eggs and tell me if you ever want to eat again!

If leptin does not elevate after a meal, serotonin will remain depressed in the brain, and cravings will ensue.

> **Diabetics should run from high-fructose corn syrup like a thief in the night, because this processed sugar is keeping you hungry for junk food, robbing you of the power to lose weight and control appetite and blood sugar. This means be wary of soda and baked goods, and check labels to ensure what you're eating has *none* of this sugar.**

Refined flour, especially when combined with saturated fat as it often is in pizza, nachos, cheeseburgers, French fries, and baked goods, sends insulin sky high. High insulin levels make you fat. Insulin shuts down all hormones responsible for using fat for fuel, and activates all hormones responsible for laying down fat. The above foods are not exactly low in calories, so guess how most of those calories are going to be stored when you eat them? Will they go toward muscle or fat? Diabetics must beware all foods with refined flour, whether or not saturated fat is present. The excessive insulin levels will provoke fat gain for hours after the meal, even keeping insulin levels elevated for days after. In short, refined flour keeps you in a fat-storing mode and away from naturally recovering from diabetes.

White sugar elevates blood sugar, spiking insulin, which then brings blood sugar back down very quickly. Even if you don't get clinically low blood sugar after the sugar rush, the rapidly swinging high and then low blood sugar will leave you craving food. When blood sugar is low, or has dropped quickly from high to low, your cravings for food will be so powerful that it will be very, very hard for you to stop eating after having only a reasonable amount. The insulin spike will have already cheated you out of losing weight for several hours after the meal, and the following cravings will set you up for a binge that can set your weight loss back days or weeks. Again, that is no way to lose weight or recover naturally from diabetes.

> **As a diabetic, you must be cautious of the quality of carbohydrates you put in your body – it's not just how many carbs or calories you eat – it's whether those carbs and calories make you then want to eat more or less.**

In the case of ingesting fructose syrup, refined flour, or sugar, they provoke you to want to eat more and more, and are therefore the most fattening. Is that hard to believe? Ask yourself if it's easier to eat 500 calories worth of white bread or Russian rye – the dark brown bread that feels like a brick in your hand. Ask yourself what's more filling – two regular sodas or eight apples. They both have the same number of calories. The lesson is clear – you create your near future appetite by what you eat next. Avoiding these foods will go a long way toward annihilating emotional eating, and ridding yourself of your greatest hindrance to weight loss – unplanned, excessive, poor-quality snacking.

Although I don't know whether my own brain was experiencing the same "neurochemical changes" as in the study above, I do know I struggled with quitting my emotional eating for years. Prior to learning I had diabetes I would have multiple several-thousand-calorie carb binges every week. They were almost always triggered by either anxiety or boredom, making them a prime example of emotional eating. And I always went for the same type of food: something high in carbohydrates. For example, I was worried about a midterm my sophomore year of college, so I ate a gallon of ice cream with chocolate syrup. When I was twenty-one, I panicked over another midterm, and ate two bear claws and a jelly doughnut with milk as a snack. I passed out shortly afterward and woke up later that evening, when my friends woke me to get drunk. Once upon a time when I was bored at work, I ate the Ben & Jerry's Cookie Dough Sundae, the Brownie Sundae, a large brownie on the side, and then a giant burrito wrap half the size of a football. Once again, I passed out immediately and woke up about three hours later. I was self-medicating my stress, anxiety, and depression with food.

Food was my personal Xanax, Prozac, and vodka cocktail, and that didn't go away even after I started to lose weight. The ability of HFCS, sugar, and refined flour to lay on fat and stir cravings became the most apparent to me when I started a low-carb diet, which reduced my binges by 80%, from about ten per month down to two. All of a sudden, I wasn't ingesting any of those bad carbs, but I was stuck in a loop: losing and then regaining the same fifteen pounds. I was exercising daily, and watching what I ate, and not making any progress. The problem was that I was still emotionally and physically attached to those high-carb foods as the study above suggested. I was simply binging on low-carb versions of ice cream, chocolate, and candy bars. I was effectively following the diabetes diet, while hanging on to my emotional addiction for carbohydrates. I was eating a low carb diet, while still finding a way to kill myself.

You don't even need a low-carb diet to kill off the above killer carbs from your diet. Fortunately, the food industry has made it very easy for you to identify which foods are the sources of emotional eating. With practice, there is little need to look at labels to find foods that will not set you off on a sugar binge. Sugar and high-fructose corn syrup are usually found in the sugar-and fat-craving foods, which can be dubbed the Eight Cs: candy, cake, cereal, chips, cola, cookies, crackers, & (ice) cream. Refined flour is often found in the fat, salt, and protein cravings – the bun on the burger, the tortilla chip, or the flour in pizza. Even brown dough can be refined, basically forcing you to read the label to be sure in this case. Avoiding these foods as much as possible will allow weight loss and stable blood sugar as quickly as possible. Removing these foods from your diet is removing the greatest negative effect to your health, leaving plenty of room in your diet for some fruits, vegetables, nuts, seeds, legumes, eggs, dairy, grains, meat, fish, and fowl.

If the dough, chip, cake or bread
is white, it's not all right.

You now understand how sugar and fat cravings can be perpetuated, and why they arise in the first place. There's nothing really wrong with having these cravings – how we solve them is the problem. Sugar and fat cravings are usually solved by bingeing on ice cream or candy bars, but why wouldn't berries with cream suffice? That question is rhetorical – it would.

> **When I learned to appease my cravings using authentic natural foods while still avoiding the killer carbohydrates, the rest of my cravings disappeared.**

Now they only reappear when I skip meals, have too much caffeine, or use too many artificial sweeteners. Fortunately, these are all things I can control. They don't control me. The remainder of this chapter is dedicated to teaching you that very same method of control.

- You can be addicted to carbohydrates. Therefore, you must take your emotional eating as a serious threat to your health, because it is the number one detrimental action you take that stands in the way of losing weight and controlling diabetes.
- Science has shown that an abnormality in neu-rotransmitters like serotonin, dopamine, and various hormones affects our willingness and even need to eat foods that are high in carbohydrates.[10-12]
- The three killer carbohydrates are high-fructose corn syrup, sugar, and refined or enriched white flour.
- The Eight Cs: candy, cake, cereal, chips, cola, cook-ies, crackers, & (ice) cream make up most of the sugar and fat cravings.
- Look through your refrigerator, pantry, and freezer. Look at the labels and notice which foods have high-fructose corn syrup, fructose syrup, corn syrup, or sugar. Start cutting back on these foods with the goal of eliminating them altogether within sixty days from now. Have one soda instead of two per day, and one candy bar every other day instead of every day. Set a goal every week to cut down a little bit more.

- Find all the foods in your home with refined, enriched, bleached, or white flour on the label. Start
  with breads, pastas, pastries, cakes, cookies, frozen
  entreés. Throw these foods out, and replace them
  only with products that have the phrase "whole
  wheat" on the label. Do one experiment first though
  – check your blood sugar an hour after eating the
  refined flour food, and an hour after the whole grain
  replacement food. What do you notice?
- How often do you crave foods high in sugar and
  fat? Do you notice any stress, anxiety, depression, or
  boredom before eating these foods?
- Overeating low-carb sweets is not the same as following a low-carb diet, or any diet for that matter.
- We diabetics all have one tremendous weakness: the
  tendency to become addicted to, and even emotionally dependent on, high-starch and high-sugar foods.

> **Changing what we eat does reduce emotional
> eating, but it takes more than that to
> ultimately quit. We create our overeating
> through our thoughts and actions, and we
> need new thoughts and actions to stop.**

Putting It Together: Your Second Prescription

As you've learned, most emotional eating comes from a
complicated chemical process that starts with being overworked,
underrested, and poorly fed. Willpower against cravings is
important, but is only part of the solution. Controlling the factors
that cause the cravings is the rest. Therefore, the best way to
control emotional eating, and to control your diabetes, is to:

- Control stress
- Get enough sleep

- Stay away from environments filled with the foods that tempt you
- Eat filling, healthy meals on a self-imposed schedule

Weight loss then happens from the day-to-day act of *not* having as many binges, pasta feeds, candy raids, and sodas as you did in the past. The more weight you lose, the more in control you'll be of your diabetes.

While you may expect recovery from emotional eating to take years, the power to instantly eliminate a food craving, no matter how strong, is readily available, and takes seconds to execute. In fact, most of the actions that control diabetes also control emotional eating. So to control emotional eating, you'll need to take your first prescription below.

Get enough sleep. Say you're a typical American with too much on your plate. You perform your daily juggling act with work, kids, bills, traffic, and your significant other. Your main concern isn't your waistline, but rather the finish line as you race to get everything done, only to start over at 5:45 AM the next day. But if your strategy for success starts with cutting back on sleep, that can be likened to shooting yourself in the foot before running a marathon. It's setting yourself up for failure.

Short of starting your day by pouring beer on your Honey Nut Cheerios, lack of sleep is the most guaranteed fat-gaining activity in your life. In fact, it might beat the Cheerios with beer. A recent study of over 1,000 individuals found that those who slept the least weighed the most. In another study, fourteen healthy young adults who slept more than seven and a half hours per night were compared to thirteen healthy young adults who slept less than six and a half hours per night. The light sleepers needed 50% more insulin to process meals and were 167% more insulin resistant after only eight days![13] Imagine how that translates if you're already diabetic!

> **Even an hour of lost sleep a few times
> a week can cause weight gain.**

There's a very simple cause and effect process going on here. Lack of sleep increases cortisol levels tremendously, which causes an increase in hunger. Poor sleepers tend to eat 15% more calories per day than people who sleep soundly.[14] Remember that cortisol is your master stress hormone, and the more stress you have, the more cravings you tend to have. Since sleep deprivation also hinders the thyroid, the gland responsible for your metabolic rate, you'll burn fewer calories if you're losing sleep. Additionally growth hormones (GH) peak in the middle of the night; this is where most people burn their fat. It's actually fat mobilized from GH that sustains you during the night, when you're not taking in any calories. If you're not maintaining a healthy sleep schedule, you can kiss the best opportunity to burn fat good-bye. Lack of sleep also lowers leptin levels in the brain, lowering serotonin. As we've seen, lower serotonin levels increase carbohydrate cravings, and that increases the drive toward emotional eating.

The end result on your metabolism and appetite is pretty abysmal. You've decreased how many calories you burn and increased how many calories you want. That means you'll be looking for five tacos at lunch. You may feel that hungry, but do you really think your metabolism is burning that much? Sleep deprivation has caused your appetite to be out of sync with your metabolic rate!

> **Most adults need around eight hours of sleep
> a night. You may need more or less than that,
> but that eight hours is a good place to start.**

If you're having trouble sleeping, and experiencing fatigue during the day, it'll affect your health. Seek help from a sleep expert, or consult your doctor. Do not compromise on this.

- When you sleep less, you crave carbs more, have

greater insulin resistance, and a slower metabolism. Is it really a wonder why this is correlated with diabetes?

• It is critical that you establish a regular bedtime, and value it over late-night television or office work.

> **Quality sleep is the first step toward taking control of your diabetes by ending emotional eating.**

Eliminate all sources of refined carbohydrates and high-fructose corn syrup from your diet. As you're learned, HFCS, sugar, and enriched flour cause nothing but food cravings and fat gain. These are ingredients that weren't even created until the twentieth century; corn syrup and white flour can only be found in a can, box, or bag. Never in nature, always in junk food. Look at the containers of sodas, snack foods, breads, pastas, and desserts in your home. If you see the words "enriched wheat flour, refined flour, corn syrup, fructose syrup, or high-fructose corn syrup (HFCS)" anywhere in the ingredients, have a Boston Tea Party with it. Just use a trash can instead of the Boston Harbor. If you're serious about controlling diabetes, weight gain, fatigue, and emotional eating, you'll get rid of these man-made foodstuffs. This is the second assignment within this prescription. It means ditching the cookies, cakes, chips, colas, candies, crackers, chocolates, cereals, croissants, and ice cream. (Croissants are in there to remind you to stay away from bread, especially white bread.)

> **Nature's versions of carbohydrates create much less blood sugar, requiring less insulin to process compared to the killer carbs.**

What carbs *can* you have? Fruits, vegetables, legumes, and some grain and dairy in their natural unrefined form. The ultimate result of this drastic change is significantly less emotional eating, weight loss, and stable blood sugar. To qualify, fruit has to be raw, not made into juice or jam. Vegetables can't be covered with 1,000 calories of salad dressing. Legumes can't be sliced into rectangles, fried, and consumed alongside a double cheeseburger. Yogurt must be plain, with unsweetened berries and Stevia, natural sweetener made from leaves, added for flavor. Grains should be whole, brown, and unrefined. Notice that this was the state of all food on the planet before the twentieth century, when type II diabetes was absolutely unheard of. This is not a coincidence. That advice may be hard to swallow, but consider that you'll read the same thing in a dozen different top sellers on health and diabetes! Even books that don't agree, agree on this.

This is an extremely important part of the program I'm prescribing for you. Your doctor cannot give you a drug that will do more for your weight loss, diabetes, and energy at the same time. Every time you eat junk, you'll want something similar within 90 to 120 minutes. You'll be craving fried chicken two hours after a Snickers and Coke. Crappy food triggers crappy cravings. Good food triggers good cravings. Simply avoiding these killer carbs can dramatically slow the progression of diabetes. You owe it to yourself to eat better.

- Enriched carbs and HFCS are linked to diabetes, obesity, and binge eating.
- The killer carbs can be found in cookies, cakes, chips, colas, candies, crackers, chocolates, cereals, croissants, and ice cream.
- Choose unaltered, natural versions of high-quality carbohydrates to control emotional eating, weight gain, and diabetes.

Cut back on natural sources of sugar and artificial sweeteners, and don't overstimulate any one of your five taste buds. Cutting artificial foods is a good first step, but you have to look at how natural foods can affect your body as well. The bottom line is that it will be very hard to kick a sugar habit if you're eating tons of sugar at each meal. If you're on a low-carb diet, but drinking twelve cans of diet soda per day, you'll never be able to kick the sugar craving. Trust me, I tried it, and it doesn't work.

This part of your assignment is simple: if you're addicted to the taste of sugar, you must cut down on your intake of natural and artificially sweetened foods and drinks. Don't go on a low-carb diet but still drink four gallons of diet soda and chew two packs of sugar-free gum every day.

Replace the addictive tastes with nonaddicting ones.

If you crave sweets, eat more bitter or savory foods. Another tip is to drink tea with lemon after eating something sweet. Eat a contrasting taste after having the taste to which you are addicted. Doing so will lessen the feedback loop between your tongue and your brain, meaning you won't continue to crave the addicting taste since you'll have most recently tasted something you're not addicted to. If you have a bite of chocolate, and follow it up with some lemon-flavored tea, your tongue will not send messages to the brain asking for more chocolate, so the sweet sensation from one chocolate does not become a gluttonous guilt trip over too much of the wrong thing!

Counteract your natural cravings and they *will* subside.

- Only you know which tastes you're addicted to, and how much of those tastes you consume daily.
- If you have a problem with sugar cravings, cut out all diet sodas, sugarless gums, and artificial sweeteners.
- Pay attention to cravings for the hour after ingesting any artificial sweeteners – did you crave anything sweet afterward?
- Brush your teeth after meals instead of using mints or sugar-free gum – you won't want to eat afterward.

Follow a low-carb diet the smart way. A low-carb diet is not necessary to "cure" food addictions, but it falls naturally under the premise of controlling diabetes and carb addictions. The very act of following a low-carb diet means that you're cutting out 99% of all processed foods and sugars from your life, thereby eliminating nearly all addictive foods. The only possible loophole in this plan is eating too many artificially sweet foodstuffs, which will create the same sort of cravings you experience with naturally sweet foods. Regardless, this way of eating also barely increases blood sugar, making it the number one natural "cure" for type II diabetes.

Blood glucose is mainly created from carbohydrates. A little is more slowly made from protein, and barely any at all from fat. By reducing your carbohydrates, you'll automatically create less glucose, and need less insulin to process that glucose. You've immediately just solved both sides of the type II diabetes riddle – high glucose and high insulin levels. At the same time, with more stable blood sugar, you can expect your cravings to decrease and energy to go up. Lower insulin levels will also cause weight loss, helping you to secure a more permanent solution to your high blood sugar – eliminating excess fat. For these reasons, you won't find a better diet out there suited to helping you heal naturally from diabetes.

In later chapters, you'll learn how to safely increase your carbohydrates on weekends, holidays, or other times of your choosing. You'll basically keep your carbs very low for five to ten days, and increase them to a predetermined level for one to two days. You'll do this indefinitely without ever suffering the old consequences of high blood sugar and weight gain.

Cycling your carbs gives you a break from the regimen of low-carb eating. You'll have plenty of room on the weekends to eat fruits, whole grains, and even old favorites like pizza and cheesecake, so don't be afraid that you'll never taste cake again. That would only build cravings over time from continual denial and psychological suppression.

> **Instead, the secret is knowing when to indulge, when not to, and honestly not wanting to because you'd rather be healthy than have another serving.**

- Cut your carbohydrates to eliminate high blood sugar and high insulin levels.
- Later, you'll learn to cycle carbs to coincide with special occasions, weekends, or holidays.

Get That Junk Food Out of the House! You can't be an emotional eater on a desert island. The food has to be there to act on the desire. So throw out all of the boxes of cookies, chips, and ice cream in your house—all of it. When you want it, you'll have to want it badly enough to go to the store and just get enough for one serving. The idea is to make it as hard as possible to get at foods that you're a sucker for, and damn near impossible to get at large quantities of them.

Is that obsessive? Do your kids need that stuff? Are you concerned that they're being denied the ability to eat wasted calories with zero nutritional value like all of the other kids in America? I was a kid once, and so were you, but I was a fat kid, and I got teased a lot for it. I would have rather had no access to those foods that contributed to my weight gain than be teased by boys and ignored by girls. I can tell you that I would have preferred to have been taught to deal with life and emotions through avenues other than eating. I would have preferred being taught to eat well, even if that meant there were no Jell-O pudding pops in the freezer or McDonalds's for dinner. Sure, I didn't know that then. And neither will your children. But that's why you're a parent. You make these decisions for them. If you're reading this book, you must on some level concur.

Does your spouse need that food? That's a rhetorical question – no one needs junk food. If it was needed, it would grow on trees. Last time I checked, cocoa did, but puffed chocolate cereal didn't. Do you really want to tell me that you're going to easily resist the cookie dough ice cream in the freezer or the beer in the refrigerator after a difficult day at work? Do yourself a favor and get rid of these foods.

> **Sometimes being an adult is admitting something is stronger than you are.**

At work and other places where you have little control, you control yourself with predetermined rules for what you will allow yourself and what you will not. You then honor that decision with the full memory of why this is so important to you. If you're at a dinner party, and you've told yourself two beers are OK, don't have three. If you're at a party, and you've told yourself one piece of cake is fine, don't have two. If you've decided to stay away from it all, don't hang out by the dessert table. If you're at a business dinner where everyone is drinking and you don't want to, don't drink. Your promotion doesn't depend on it.

Keep full on fiber. Fiber slows the release of glucose into your system. A slower release of sugar into your blood ultimately means lower blood sugar. Fiber also keeps you fuller longer, and therefore goes a long way to controlling diabetes. In addition, filling up without adding calories is a major recipe for fat loss. This is why vegetables are such a great tool in a healthy diabetic's life. They're low in calories, low in carbohydrates, and extremely filling. Broccoli, cauliflower, spinach, cucumber, watercress, asparagus, and lettuce will give you something to munch on all day if you need the oral fix. Use a zero-calorie dressing if you must, but be warned that labels can report zero calories per serving if they have fewer than five. You could inadvertently consume 100 to 200 extra calories if you gorge on the dressing, so it's always best to eat veggies steamed or even raw. Better yet, sprinkle some Real Salt on them and douse them with fresh lemon.

Another choice is to use glucomannan, a tasteless, clear soluble fiber that bulks up your food, blunts insulin release, and delays hunger. Adding two to four grams of glucomannan to your eggs, cottage cheese, yogurt, chili, or smoothie will fill you up with far fewer calories. Your food will be heavy and filling, while still maintaining a low-calorie count. By adding fiber to your small frequent meals, you'll be so stuffed that you won't want to eat anything else. Again, this prevents emotional eating. You won't feel like you're missing a thing, especially those extra pounds packed on by endlessly overeating!

- Use fiber to fill up without adding calories – you'll be too full to want to emotionally eat.
- Glucomannan is the number one best fiber for bulking up food and controlling blood sugar in diabetics – women and men should get eight to twelve grams and ten to fifteen grams per day respectively.

Eat the same way day in and day out. Plan your meals, make your shopping list, buy your food, prepare it over the weekend, and maintain a schedule over the week. In other words, plan what you'll eat ahead of time, and then eat it. This doesn't mean that you have to eat boring meals every day. It means you need to find meals that are healthy, and that you'll look forward to, and make sure you stick to them.

People are creatures of habit; they eat the same types of food, day in and day out. How much variety do you incorporate in your eating? Do you have thirty different breakfasts, lunches, and dinners per month? Fifteen? Seven? The average is closer to one or two, which makes it very easy. Just make sure your one or two habitual meals are food that will help you control blood sugar, cravings, and weight gain. Then do the same thing tomorrow. It really is that simple.

The one caveat to this simplicity is the planning, which is where most people fail. They fail to plan their meals, so they fail to buy the right food, and have nothing to prep. To truly heal by controlling your eating and blood sugar, you must plan, pay, prep, and eat. Then do it again next week.

Eat five to six meals a day, one every two to three hours.
Becoming a healthy diabetic means avoiding emotional eating, which requires making good food choices every day, at every meal. And you can't make good food choices when you're ravenously hungry. Letting yourself get to that point by not planning when and what to eat ahead of time invites emotional eating into your life. Evade that trap by planning, preparing, and packing the right food. Make sure that you have enough healthy food on hand at all times, and eat it at regular intervals. This will help you avoid randomly heading to the candy machine when hunger strikes.

Small frequent meals also help keep your blood sugar more stable than large meals eaten six hours apart.[15, 16] Remember that when blood sugar is at a happy medium, neither too high nor too low, hunger will be less and energy and mood will be higher. Insulin levels will be optimally low, and serotonin will not come crashing down. Eating frequent small meals also keeps your appetite low, because you're either eating or digesting food for the entire day. That's another preventative strategy against emotional eating that you won't get from big meals spaced far apart from each other.

So when will you eat? You have to know that in advance to put this plan into action. First, decide when you'll eat breakfast, ensuring it's within an hour of rising. Next, schedule the rest of the meals, each spaced two to three hours apart from each other, depending on when you tend to become hungriest and what fits your schedule best.

If you're accustomed to eating two or three large meals in a day, or even skipping breakfast, you may not be that hungry in the early morning. If that's the case, you should force something down like a hard-boiled egg or a few slices of cheese until you begin to naturally eat earlier in the day. As you start to become a breakfast eater, you'll naturally find your evening appetite diminishing as your body becomes accustomed to metabolizing calories earlier rather than later. As a bonus, your evening cravings will diminish. This is generally when cravings are at their worst, but not for you, not anymore.

Split the size of your typical first meal of the day in half, and eat half for breakfast and half for brunch. Do the same with lunch, eating half at noon and half in the early afternoon. Have a smaller dinner, and if hungry, a light snack a few hours later. Stop eating within two hours of bedtime so your digestion does not interfere with your sleep.

Each meal should have a serving of protein and fiber and be devoid of high-fructose corn syrup, sugar, and refined flour. For breakfast, try one of these:

- Three eggs scrambled in coconut oil (cooking oil) with glucomannan powder mixed in for fiber (300 calories and 1 carb)
- Three cheese sticks and ¼ cup of almonds (400 calories and 5 carbs)
- A protein shake with milled flaxseeds, fish oil, vanilla extract, and frozen berries (300 calories and 7 carbs)
- Try the following snacks over your usual high-in-sugar and fat snacks at brunch and midafternoon:
- A small pear with two string cheeses (160 calories and 10 carbs)
- ½ cup low fat cottage cheese with ¼ cup sliced almonds and ¼ cup blackberries (300 calories and 15 carbs)
- ½ cup low fat cottage cheese with 1 tablespoon almond butter, 1 tablespoon raw cocoa and one packet of Stevia (240 calories and 7 carbs)
- Lunch and dinner could look like the following:
- 6 ounces broiled salmon with steamed vegetables (400 calories and 5 carbs)
- 6 ounce salmon filet with steamed vegetables (400

calories and 5 carbs)

- Chef salad with light dressing (500 calories and 5 carbs)

Choose tea over coffee to prevent cravings from too much caffeine, and brush your teeth between meals instead of using gum or breath mints. Stevia is the only natural noncaloric sweetener, so it's the only acceptable sweetener. Reorganizing your meals while cutting out the carbs, caffeine, and artificial sweeteners will dramatically reduce your blood sugar over time. You may notice an increase in cravings over the first two weeks of starting this new regime due to physical withdrawals from sugar and caffeine. It will all pass. Once the withdrawals are gone, you'll have more energy, less hunger, and fewer cravings. You'll have taken a huge step in controlling your diabetes and your life.

- Decide when you'll eat all six meals, starting with breakfast.
- Eat half of what you normally do for breakfast, lunch, and dinner, and add snacks between.
- Cut your carbs, ensuring there is no high-fructose corn syrup, refined flour, or sugar in your meals.
- Have protein and fiber at every meal.
- Substitute tea for coffee, and only use Stevia for a sweetener.

Wait out the cravings. Ghrelin, the hunger hormone in the stomach, will remain elevated and induce hunger when stimulated, meaning that if you wait it out, ghrelin will lower, tell NPY to go lower, and the physical and mental desire to eat will subside. The solution to the symptom here is to wait it out! Stay away from all food and sources of this food for one hour. Afterward, the desire will be lessened.

The long-term solution to the root of the problem is of course to lose weight and control your blood sugar. I have found that my food cravings are *far* less than what they used to be. There is light at the end of the tunnel. As Winston Churchill once said, "If you're going through hell, keep going."

Take supplements that alleviate cravings. There are supplements that can safely boost serotonin in the brain to fight cravings. You may recall that the amino acid tryptophan is used to create serotonin. Specifically, tryptophan is converted to 5-Hydroxytryptophan (5-HTP) before finally being converted into serotonin. So it makes intuitive sense that increasing your intake of tryptophan or 5-HTP will increase serotonin levels in your brain. We've already seen that increasing serotonin levels leads to less hunger, better sleep, stable mood, and fewer carbohydrate cravings. As I previously stated, this is why Prozac and other SSRIs are prescribed to treat emotional eating. Ironically, they also cause weight gain. Isn't avoiding weight gain at the heart of 99% of everyone taking an SSRI to quit emotionally eating? What's also not commonly discussed are the studies that have shown that 5-HTP is as effective as Prozac and other SSRIs in yielding the above benefits.[17] Naturally speaking, 5-HTP is actually a more direct route to those benefits. Instead of artificially blocking brain chemicals that destroy serotonin to keep more of it in the brain as SSRIs do, 5-HTP naturally triggers serotonin. With serotonin on your side, you get satisfaction from meals, resistance to carbohydrate cravings, and a willingness to voluntarily eat less. And it's also cheaper, safer, available without a prescription, and relatively void of side effects.[18] This is by far the more natural prescription, and one that you can control yourself.

Facts about 5-HTP have been proven by several scientific studies. Scientists who gave 3.5 milligrams of 5-HTP per pound of body weight to obese females found that it helped the subjects decrease food intake and lose weight, without affecting their mood (as Prozac does).[20] In another study, scientists fed 900 milligrams of 5-HTP per day to twenty obese subjects for twelve weeks. The study was split into two six-week time spans. The subjects were told to eat as much as they wanted for the first six weeks, and then given a 1,200-calorie limit for the second six weeks. Compared to the control group, those who were given 5-HTP voluntarily ate fewer carbs, were more quickly satisfied by their meals, and lost more weight.[21] Such studies validate that 5-HTP supplementation is a very safe and effective method for you to naturally increase serotonin, increase satisfaction from food, and beat emotional eating.

A 5-HTP supplement can be taken with meals without reducing its effectiveness. Over half of it will eventually be converted into straight serotonin[17] instead of wasted by the body over various metabolic processes. An effective dosage for appetite control is 3.5 milligrams per pound of body weight, split into two or three dosages throughout the day. Although you can take it with meals, taking it thirty minutes prior to meals is actually more beneficial; the presence of more serotonin will optimize your resistance to cravings and actually increase satiety from the forthcoming meal. In short, you'll probably eat less.

- To fight sugar and fat cravings, multiply your body weight by 3.5, divide that by 3, and then take that many milligrams of 5-HTP three times per day, thirty minutes before meals.

L-glutamine, an amino acid found in nearly 70% of your muscle, can also instantly kill your sugar cravings.[24] This supplement supplies your brain with immediate energy, which halts the process that leads to cravings. It also binds with your sweet taste buds, "satisfying" their desire for stimulation. Place ten grams of L-glutamine powder in a sixteen-ounce bottle of water, and take two large sips with each craving. If you get a craving, take a sip and watch the craving disappear. If you get another craving later, take another sip. Think of L-glutamine like pouring water on an emotional-eating fire – it puts out the flames. One caveat about looking for glutamine powder online or in a health food store—don't mistake L-glutamine for glutamine peptide – they're completely different.

- To immediately end sugar cravings, consume two grams of L-glutamine powder.
- To avoid sugar cravings as they arise over the day, place ten grams of L-glutamine in sixteen ounces of water, and drink about one-fifth of the bottle for each

craving (equating to two grams of L-glutamine).

Gymnema sylvestre, an ayurvedic herb used in India for thousands of years, also decreases carbohydrate cravings. It has a bitter taste due to the herb's high content in Gymnemic acids, which have an anti-sweet effect. So placing Gymnema sylvestre on the tongue kills the craving for sugar by creating a feedback loop going from your sweet taste buds to your brain. The herb also helps emotional eating by improving insulin sensitivity, the cell's ability to use insulin efficiently.[25] The more sensitive your cells are to taking up insulin from the blood, the more nutrients and blood sugar can be used by them. Since less insulin is needed by the cells to process glucose and nutrients, it is far less likely to accumulate in the blood to the point that your blood sugar drops very fast, causing a blood sugar crash and carb cravings. Take 100 mg three times per day, or whenever you feel cravings coming on.

- 5-HTP is converted into serotonin and can be used to decrease sugar and fat cravings. Take 3.5 mg per pound of body weight divided into three doses each day thirty minutes before eating.
- Two grams of L-glutamine can immediately curb sugar cravings.
- 100 mg of Gymnema sylvestre can also kill sugar cravings.

Know when you're susceptible!

It's natural to become hungry and tired at midmorning and midafternoon thanks to dipping cortisone levels. Millions of years of evolution have caused our bodies to have the greatest lull in cortisone levels over a twenty-four hour period at approximately 10 AM and 2 PM, not coincidentally the times that are famous for coffee breaks and siestas around the world. By having a snack before these two lulls in the

**day, you'll keep your serotonin and energy
levels up, and avoid the temptation to snack on
sweets and onion rings with your coworkers.**

Cortisone helps the liver to release glycogen, a fancy word for chains of carbohydrate. This increase in blood sugar is usually a good thing that prevents blood sugar from dropping too low. However, this drop in cortisone at midmorning and midafternoon means blood sugar and serotonin levels will both go lower, increasing the potential for emotional eating. Diabetic or not, this one-two punch leaves you feeling lethargic, unfocused, and hungry. This is when the body will start specifically craving carbs. This is also the danger zone for a diabetic: giving in to carb cravings now will start a downward cycle of blood sugar highs and lows throughout the day. Eat before that happens.

Most people get their worst cravings at night. If you need a high-carb feast to sleep, skimp on breakfast, and eat most of your calories at night, you probably have nighttime eating syndrome (NES). To be blunt, this is emotional eating hell. If eating small, frequent, and high-protein meals is the eating style of the lean, then eating large, late, and high-carb meals is the eating style of the obese. The latter style has less to do with preference and more to do with brain chemistry. Years of eating foods high in sugar and fat can disrupt leptin levels, the hormone excreted from your fat cells that controls metabolism. Regulating the metabolism doesn't stop at determining how many calories you burn or how much fat you carry – it also includes when you're hungry and for what. Overeating high-carb meals laden with sugar and fat causes too much leptin to be excreted, which over time causes the brain to become less and less sensitive to leptin levels. This turns into a leptin resistance, which ultimately results in a feast or famine state in the body – you're not hungry at all in the morning, but very hungry at night. Unfortunately, that hunger is for all the wrong foods – meals very high in sugar and fat to shoot leptin through the roof at night, stay elevated in the morning hours, but then drop again in the evening hours. When leptin drops, cravings ensue. Why is this so bad for weight gain?

> **Having a metabolism that wants to starve itself for half the day, but then overfeed itself for the other half is like yo-yo dieting to the body – you're going to gain more and more weight over time because you ultimately eat more calories than you burn in a day eating this way.**

As you've already read, high-carb meals also screw up your serotonin levels, also adding to the cravings. Therefore, if you eat most of your food at night and little or nothing for breakfast, you've locked yourself into a fat-gaining trap.

You'll need to reset your body's internal clock so it wants to eat *more* in the morning and *less* in the evening. For this reason, melatonin and 5-HTP are the NES sufferer's best friends. Melatonin is a hormone excreted by the pineal gland between your eyes that is responsible for inducing sleep. It's actually the next step in serotonin's neurochemical evolution – tryptophan converts to 5-HTP, then serotonin, and finally melatonin. For reasons not yet entirely understood by scientists, 0.5 to 3 mg of melatonin have been shown to help NES sufferers overcome their problems with leptin[2], the devilish little hormone that worked with serotonin to ruin your life. The reason likely has to do with melatonin inducing sleep – when you have NES, you usually can't sleep until you've had a huge carb binge to increase serotonin and melatonin in the brain. By directly supplementing with melatonin, your brain achieves one of its two goals without needing 500 grams of sugar to achieve it. Supplementing with 100 to 300 mg of 5-HTP at night takes care of the other goal. As a result, you'll be able to avoid the huge carb cravings, allowing you to eat less at night, creating more hunger in the morning, all the while bringing leptin back to where it should be.

At night, eat a high-protein, high-fiber dinner to fend off late-night snacking. Protein and fiber at dinner will keep you full throughout the night, and help you fight the infamous diabetic midnight munchies. You'll wake up feeling healthier, ready to face the day with a balanced blood sugar level, rather than recovering from your midnight binge. Your blood sugar will be more stable the next day thanks to how well you took care of yourself the previous night.

To reinforce this idea, whether you want to or not, you should also absolutely force yourself to eat breakfast and lunch at the very beginning. It's the only way you'll become hungry in the AM instead of the PM. Eventually, you'll never know how you were able to skip breakfast and eat so much at night. When that happens, you've successfully recovered from NES. You'll have eliminated the greatest cause of late-night eating, eliminated a source of fat gain, and helped to bring your blood sugar back under control.

- The bottom line – know when you'll be hungry during the day, and eat before that happens.
- Eating your biggest meal at night while not being able to fall asleep without ingesting a ton of carbs may be a sign of nighttime eating disorder. 5-HTP and Melatonin can help this.
- If you're experiencing cravings after a healthy meal, try a low-calorie treat (good), small taste of whatever you're craving (better), or wait it out (best). This usually occurs at night, in the danger time.
- Schedule your frequent small meals with your most susceptible times for cravings in mind. For most people, that will be midmorning, midafternoon, and dinnertime.

Stop using food as a coping mechanism by learning other ways to deal with your cravings. So far, you've learned to reduce cravings and stop them from ever appearing. The techniques covered all attack emotional eating from the brain's perspective. Now we will attack it from the mind's. In the Eleventh Prescription, you'll learn the following five-step technique to identify the root of your emotional eating and eliminate it.

1. Know that you can have that food any time.
2. Don't block or withhold any thoughts about that food. Savor it, smell it, and remember how good it tastes.
3. At this point, ask yourself these four questions about the food you're craving.
   a. What do you believe is the value of eating that food?
   b. How do you feel when eating that food?
   c. What do you think is the reason you should eat that food?
   d. What are your behaviors given this desire for this food, beyond whether or not you decide to eat it?
4. Now ask yourself these four questions about eating healthy food instead.
   a. What do you believe is the value of eating healthy portions of healthy food?
   b. How do you feel about eating healthy portions of healthy food?
   c. What do you think is the reason to eat healthy portions of healthy food?
   d. What are your behaviors around eating healthy portions of healthy food, beyond whether or not you follow through?
5. Now decide without guilt if you would rather eat the food you crave, or stay the course with your healthy eating. Most important, you must be completely comfortable with either choice.

Going through these five steps reveals where, when, why, and how you emotionally eat.

Increasing serotonin is not just about popping serotonin boosters and learning better eating habits. By actively changing your normal response to stress and anxiety using the above technique, you can save yourself millions of calories over your lifetime to prevent dozens of pounds of fat. But that's not the only way to ward off stress. For example, one of the easiest ways to boost serotonin and relieve stress is to take a nap. If luxury affords, take one when stressed! You're really not going to have as much desire for cheesecake after doing so.

If work is making you stressed, then take more breaks. Yes, take more breaks, because it will make you more productive, not less. As outlined by Jim Loehr and Tony Schwartz in *The Power of Full Engagement*, research shows that the human body and mind are more productive if sixty to ninety minutes of focused attention is followed by a ten- to twenty-minute break.[26] They give very practical evidence that managing your energy, not your time, is how to become as productive and invigorated as possible with the least perceived stress. When you watch a half hour less of television to sleep another half hour, increasing productivity and decreasing cravings the next day, you just managed your energy without creating more time. When you take a break at work that refreshes you so you can get more done in less time, you just managed energy. When you're working very well, you're experiencing little to no cravings. The reason is it's impossible for the brain to work optimally if it's depleted in key neurotransmitters like serotonin or dopamine, and cravings *will* happen if you're deficient in either of these. So by managing your energy to optimize your performance at work, you are by definition optimizing your brain's chemicals, simultaneously decreasing cravings. The two go hand in hand.

Managing energy is at the heart of managing emotional eating.

Applying these techniques above should be done alongside all the other strategies learned thus far to control emotional eating. By attacking the problem from mind, body, and brain's perspective, you cover every way that emotional eating creeps up on you. With this problem under control, you'll be able to stick to a way of eating that allows you to control blood sugar and lose weight, the only real "cure" for type II diabetes.

Control your blood sugar. Of course if it was that easy, you wouldn't need this book. Controlling blood sugar controls insulin. By preventing highs and lows in blood sugar via proper diet and exercise, you prevent needing extra insulin from an injection, via a pill, or your own pancreas. Needing less insulin in effect means blood sugar neither goes too high nor too low. By preventing blood sugar from going too high, you prevent all the consequences of diabetes. Likewise, by preventing blood sugar from going too low, you prevent craving sugar and carbs.

> **The heart of diabetes is the body's inability to use the insulin it has, so you must eliminate your emotional eating as the first step in helping it take up insulin properly, thereby controlling your blood sugar for good. And if you can learn to control your blood sugar, you'll have fewer cravings, less often.**

As you move through this program and start to take control, expect your cravings to naturally subside. You'll have fewer lulls, and fewer sugar binges. With fewer sugar binges come fewer highs. With fewer highs come fewer rebounding lulls. The emotional eating cycle – caused by both your mind and your body – will be broken.

Emotionally eating can also come directly from medications for diabetes that brings your blood sugar *too* low, causing hypoglycemia. I've had this happen to me even when taking Metformin, a prescription medication for diabetes that is not usually expected to cause low blood sugar! Once you can control this disease without swallowing pills or injecting shots (or as few as possible), you won't crash as often, which will go a long way to controlling emotional eating even better. So here's how we've learned to control emotional eating.

> **Control blood sugar, and you control emotional eating. Control emotional eating, and you control blood sugar.**

The Second Prescription in Summary

- Emotional eating is the spark that lights the diabetic dynamite. You have to have the genes to get this disease, but our behaviors turn that potential into reality.
- Emotional eating is defined through its excessiveness. It's eating to satisfy cravings other than the body's needs regardless of how good it tastes.
- Knowing why you emotionally eat is the key to being able to follow a healthy diet long term. Following a healthy diet long term is the cornerstone to losing weight and getting diabetes under control.
- The two key cravings are for sugar and fat together or fat, protein, and salt together. The former is caused by low serotonin, the latter by low dopamine.
- Both types of cravings come about from stress, lack of sleep, too much caffeine, and, most important, eating foods high in refined flour and sugar. Our food creates our cravings.
- Completely cut out high-fructose corn syrup, refined four, and processed sugar from your diet. Throw out foods with these ingredients on the label.
- Get enough sleep each night without exception.
- Eat five to six times per day, once every two to three hours, making breakfast your largest meal and dinner the smallest.

- Have a serving of protein and fiber at every meal.
- Supplement with 5-HTP, L-glutamine, & Gymnema sylvestre to fight food cravings.
- Use extra 5-HTP and melatonin at night if you suspect nighttime eating syndrome.
- Follow a low-carb diet.
- Use Stevia as your only artificial sweetener, and cut out diet soda. No more Equal, Splenda, or Sweet'n Low. Brush your teeth instead of using breath mints or gum.
- Take breaks from work every sixty to ninety minutes.
- Nap in the afternoon when you can.

Don't Let Craving Sugar Mean High Blood Sugar

Emotional eating is like holding your breath between meals. When cravings arrive, you hyperventilate. Like breathing, the trick is to learn to take food in sips instead of giant gulps. It doesn't work to be good for six days with your eating and then binge on the seventh day. You wouldn't tell an addict to stay drug free on the weekdays, but have all the cocaine he wanted on Saturday. Days and days of being good will not cancel out the damage done to your weight and blood sugar by a one-day all-out binge. You will have to learn moderation with all foods.

> **If you want to control your diabetes, you need to learn a very powerful lesson: 20% of your success will come from what you put in your mouth. The other 80% will come from what you don't.**

By not putting junk food in your mouth—by not emotionally eating—you can start losing weight and controlling blood sugar. You want to remove this negative in your life while you work on positives like exercise.

Emotional eaters use food as a drug, but recovering is not like quitting cocaine. Abstinence is not possible. You must learn to eat in a way that does not exacerbate diabetes or weight gain.

Fortunately, life will offer you an almost unlimited number of practice sessions to get it right. Every deadline you have to meet, every time your friends invite you to a bar, and every time you go out on a date – they're all opportunities to adopt a new response to a familiar situation. This doesn't mean you can't celebrate with dinner and cheesecake anymore. It does mean you can't have cheesecake *for* dinner.

The strategies you've learned so far will annihilate most of your sugar and fat cravings if you use them. However, stress can still rear its ugly head and make emotional eating a living hell by causing cravings for high-calorie salty foods. The third prescription will arm you with the tools to deal with the other type of classic craving. Once armed, you'll be able to stick to the *New Diabetes Prescription's* eating plan without falling off the wagon, having to get back on again, and again, and again.

*All stress-induced weight gain can be sidestepped simply by realizing that you have some control over **your stressors, and total control over how you respond to them.***"

THIRD PRESCRIPTION

Change the Stress, or Change Your Response

*T*his tip is so important, so involved, that it deserves its own chapter. So I gave it one. In the previous chapter, you learned how to stop sugar and fat cravings caused by low serotonin. In this chapter, you'll learn how to solve stress-induced depletion of dopamine, which causes cravings for protein, fat, and salt together like that found in pizza, nachos, and cheeseburgers. And while a day of stress may only cause the occasional pizza craving, when you have a life full of stress, you gain weight like it's always the holiday season. As mentioned in the First Prescription, chronic stress leaves cortisone, the stress hormone, elevated all day long increasing insulin resistance. It also causes adrenaline resistance, blunting fat gain and exacerbating cravings further. And it only gets worse as our work hours increase, our relaxation drops, and our access to fattening foods grows.

It shouldn't be that hard for you even now to understand the strong connection between stress and poor health. Just picture all the bad habits that gravitate around managing stress. As you'll learn, overeating and using stimulants excessively make fat loss harder by overloading your system, and making fat loss harder makes controlling blood sugar harder. Therefore, to control diabetes, you have to change the way you deal with stress, and you have to create less of it.

A Tale of Stress Making You Fatter and More Diabetic

We've all had deadlines at work, those projects where you come to work two hours early and stay four hours late. You put your personal life on hold. Sometimes you even put your hygiene on hold (hey, it happens). Nerves are touchy. People are cranky. But there's no sign of relief until the project is finished, the deadline weeks or even months away. Even under this kind of pressure, most people are able to maintain some sort of equilibrium – less sleep and fewer breaks, but nevertheless you rationalize that if you maintain this pace, you'll be able to make it to the finish line with your sanity.

And then you get the e-mail. Or the phone call. Or the visit from your coworker with the look on her face that can only mean one thing. This job is now going to suck, and the only thing that is going to suck more than this job will be my life until this hell is *over*.

This is when those reserves in your stamina come into play. You feel the sweat on your forehead and collar. You really wish business casual included shorts on days like this. You're rushing between the printer and your desk. Your pulse is racing. There's a knot in your solar plexus. You're speed walking to your boss's office for approval on the next section. Your heart is now pounding, and your pupils are half their normal size. While on the phone, you tap your fingers for every two seconds that you're on hold. Everything takes too much time, and there isn't enough time for anything. This is the danger time – you can't stop working, but you need to do *something* to release the tension. For a lot of people, diabetic or not, this means stress cravings...

It's been ninety minutes since this crisis started and you're already wearing thin. For some odd reason, that sandwich that normally keeps you full until at least 4:30 isn't protecting you from the leftover birthday cake in the fridge. You're not hungry, per se, but you're desperately craving the taste of sugar in your mouth. That's a craving that you would not have had if you weren't so stressed. You're actually salivating, and although your stomach is full, it's murmuring for some action. You can't get the thought of that cake out of your head. What is going on!?

Your willpower lasts five whole minutes before you cut yourself a huge slice of cake, and you pour a Coke into a plastic cup to go with it. But you rationalize that since you're having a bad day, you deserve to treat yourself. After wolfing down the snack, you get back to your desk to tackle the situation with newfound stamina and exuberance. Crisis averted, you think to yourself. But is it?

If this was the first time you'd done this, you wouldn't be so concerned about your ever-increasing blood sugar and waistline. But you've noticed that you're averaging three or four crises a month, which totals five or six such breakdowns every month. That means five or six extra sugar binges that no one can afford, never mind a diabetic trying to gain control of his or her life. Overeating is bad enough for a nondiabetic. But for anyone with diabetes or prediabetes, the consequences are worse – more weight gain and worse health.

The larger problem is that these won't be isolated incidents. As humans we are creatures of habit, and the person who runs to the candy machine every time he or she encounters stress will not be able to calmly moderate their junk food intake during the nonstressful times, when opportunities to eat badly are staring them in the face. Once a person gets on the junk food or candy train, they maintain these habits. As diabetics, we cannot afford to let our stress change the way we eat for the worst. It literally puts our health in danger.

Fortunately, all stress-induced weight gain can be sidestepped simply by realizing that *you have some control over your stressors, and total control over how you respond to them.* You can tolerate nearly any stress without changing your job, your kids, or your spouse. I hope that's the most empowering news you've learned all day, because it's the absolute truth.

The third prescription will allow you to avoid having stress in your life become stress in your body, ending the fat gain and high blood sugar roller coaster. And that stress doesn't end at overeating. Abusing caffeine, nicotine, and other stimulants are a stress to the body because they force cortisone and adrenaline levels upward when abused. Natural alternatives to these plus learning to moderate these substances in the first place will go a long way toward managing stress.

The Ingredients of the Third Prescription

The global answer to solving stress is obvious: don't overwork yourself. Everyone has a limit on the amount of stress they can deal with. Know your own, and don't tax your body beyond that. You've already learned three ways to fend off stress in the Second Prescription. The first and best way is to ensure you're getting enough rest at night.

Since sleep is the number one way the body regenerates, that is obviously key in dealing with stress. Eating frequent small meals is also nothing new. Finally, avoiding high-fructose syrup and refined sugar and flour are so important, they bear repeating. Below, you'll learn to manipulate caffeine and a few amino acids for maximum stress release and freedom from food cravings. This is a very large key to controlling your stress, thereby controlling weight gain and even diabetes.

L-theanine as a Stress Reliever

If you feel anxiety, panic, or stress at bedtime, it will affect your ability to fall asleep. As you've already learned, this can tax your energy reserves, leading to weight gain. It can also indirectly lead to blood sugar roller coasters through the day. But the solution is not Ambien or Xanax.

You don't need sleeping pills or antianxiety medication to calm down over the day or fall asleep at night. There is an amino acid that can do the job for less than a prescription copay and without side effects such as drowsiness, dizziness, lightheadedness, decreased libido, dry mouth, increased hunger, hallucinations, impaired judgment, or headaches.

If you're having trouble sleeping, it's making your diabetes and weight worse, and that makes L-theanine your new secret weapon. It's your natural Ambien and Xanax rolled into one.[1] L-theanine is an amino acid found in green tea that is responsible for its energizing, focus-enhancing, and calming effect on the body.[17] It works primarily by increasing GABA, the neurotransmitter that Xanax and other benzodiazepines bind to in order to create a relaxed and less anxious mental state. Theanine also increases serotonin levels, adding to its calming effect. The only way it can make you tired is by taking too much of it. Think of theanine as removing the anxiety, but not inducing fatigue. If it's nighttime, and you're no longer keyed up thanks to theanine, you can naturally fall asleep. However, if it's daytime, and your anxiety is impairing your work, a little theanine can remove it without making you groggy. Unlike prescription medications, you can safely and judiciously give yourself the right amount at the right time without unwanted side effects. With the right dosage, theanine will even make you more focused since it also increases dopamine levels in the brain.

Have you ever noticed that coffee gets you keyed up, whereas green tea doesn't? The reason is not due to the caffeine level, even when drinking enough green tea to match that in a sixteen-ounce cup of coffee! The reason is that L-theanine neutralizes the overstimulating effects of caffeine. It *will* relieve your anxiety and nervousness, and it will do so safely.[2]

If drinking too much caffeine gives you insomnia at night, L-theanine can still help you since it is so effective at countering stimulants. Theanine shuts down the caffeine rush that's keeping you awake by increasing GABA and serotonin.[3] If you need your caffeine during the day, but then can't sleep at night, take 100 to 200 mg of L-theanine thirty minutes before bed. Do not exceed 300 mg. You *will* fall asleep.

Like I've already said, Xanax and other benzodiazepines are not the answer for most people's stressful days at work—nor is alcohol. Both leave you mentally impaired and unable to finish your work, which sometimes is the only thing that is going to eventually end your rotten day. Meanwhile, L-theanine can be taken during the day to directly alleviate stress without making you fall asleep when you need to be at your best. Starting with a standard dosage of 50 to 200 mg taken once may be all you need. It will last for eight to twelve hours. You can also take 100 to 200 mg three times a day if stress is ongoing, but you should not exceed 1,200 mg in twenty-four hours.[3]

Relieving yourself from stress using prescription medication or overeating will leave you with more harm than good. The side effect of poor blood sugar control and weight gain from too much stress will be worse than the stress itself. Fortunately, using simple, natural solutions like theanine, you don't have to choose between feeling normal and doing something good for your health. The same choice can take care of both. Theanine is safe, effective, and natural. The next time you encounter stress or feel panicked, make it your first plan of action. You have nothing to lose but your health if you don't.

- If you regularly suffer from insomnia, wake up recurrently during the night, or have trouble getting into a deep sleep, have 1-3 mg of melatonin with 200 to 400 mg of 5-HTP one hour before bedtime.
- If caffeine or the residual stress of the day is keeping you up at night, add 200 mg of L-theanine.
- The stimulating effects of any stress, whether from a large meal, too much alcohol, or sinus medication, can usually be neutralized with theanine.

Caffeine Causes Cravings

Coffee is stress in a bean. It gives you an up and then a down, making coffee more of a loan on energy than a gift. In fact, all caffeinated beverages, fat burners, and amphetamines cause the release of the stress hormones cortisone, adrenaline, and glucagon. Recall that cortisone and adrenaline are your primary stress hormones, and glucagon is insulin's opposite. Each of these hormones leads to breakdown in liver glycogen, which you'll recall is stored carbohydrate. When done in excess, this process spikes insulin for transport of those released carbs back into your cells. In fact, whenever glucagon causes the liver to release glycogen, insulin is signaled to store that glycogen immediately. Blood glucose will enter your cells too quickly, rapidly dropping blood sugar. In the end, you'll crash as though you've just had three large bags of candy. The swinging blood sugar of a diabetic makes the low blood sugar crash and subsequent carb cravings even worse. This is why you start to feel hungry sixty to ninety minutes after a cup of coffee.

There are some studies that have shown that caffeinated coffee drinkers have a lower incidence of diabetes than noncoffee drinkers, and others that have shown that caffeine raises glucose and insulin resistance in diabetics.[18] This is an issue of science seeming to point in both directions. The best reason to avoid caffeinated coffee (and as you'll learn, drink green tea instead) is because caffeinated coffee is far more of a stress on the body than caffeinated green tea.[19-20] As you'll remember, stress increases hunger and slows metabolism. Too much cortisone for too long increases blood sugar and insulin resistance. If adrenaline resistance sets in, cravings for fat, protein, and salt and fat and sugar will go through the roof. Therefore, less stress means fewer binges. It's a difference between being hungry every 90 minutes versus being hungry every 150 minutes. It's the difference between having two pieces of candy a day versus not craving it at all. It's the difference between gaining half a pound a week versus actually losing weight. Remember, 80% of your fat loss will come from what you never put in your mouth—both directly and indirectly.

Over the last five years, replacing eight cups of water for eight cups of coffee (yes, eight!) has given me more energy, less hunger, better blood sugar control, and fewer sugar cravings. Two weeks before my last college finals, I had become so accustomed to caffeine that it was nothing more than flavored water to me. I could sleep right through a twenty-ounce cup. But I'd made a deal with myself: I wasn't about to get Bs on my finals because I couldn't stay awake, and it was worth the possible repercussions on my health. My method of stimulation was safer than that of some of the engineering and pre-med students who'd buy Ritalin from students with ADHD. Instead, I used Twinlab's Ripped Fuel, which contained both ephedrine and caffeine. I got an A+ and an A- on my two math finals. Then I paid the price with adrenaline fatigue, spending the next three months exhausted and burned out.

If you're taking fat burners or other stimulants, cut back or completely eliminate your coffee intake. You're doubling up, and causing your body twice as much stress. Remember that all stimulants are loans against the sympathetic nervous system. If you keep demanding more adrenaline and noradrenaline from your body by using stimulants, you'll pay back with interest in the form of fatigue, greater appetite, and not feeling like yourself anymore. And that loan can take as long as a year to pay back. The interest on that loan will include weight gain, excessive hunger, and cravings for foods in amounts you otherwise would not want. You will not be able to withstand the urge to comfort yourself with sugar and fat and push forward with fat, protein, and salt foods. It's better to take things slower, avoiding the trap in the first place by never overdoing it on stimulants and by *getting enough sleep*. That's the real way to have more energy during the day.

- Coffee is another stress on an already stressed diabetic body. A little is fine, but using it to stay awake instead of sleeping enough is when you start to pay a price.

- In general, it's best to limit caffeine intake to two cups of coffee, or 200 mg of caffeine per day from coffee. Note that a cup would be a small size at Starbucks.
- While 200 mg of caffeine may optimal, if you must have more, limit your total daily intake to no more than 400 to 600 mg of caffeine per day.
- A lot of stress stems from not getting enough sleep, which creates the need for coffee. However, coffee only fatigues the adrenals. It does not give energy; it lends it out with a high interest rate.
- Too much coffee diminishes cognitive performance. One study done on optimal caffeine intake showed that those who had no coffee did no better on cognitive tests than those who took 300 mg of caffeine from coffee. That's the amount of caffeine in a medium cup of coffee from most coffeehouses. Those who only took 150 mg did the best[5]. More is not better.

Green Tea: The Anti Coffee

For the gift of energy with blood sugar control plus fat loss to boot, green tea is a better choice than coffee or even fat burners. While green and black tea are likely the only two you've heard of, they are in fact derived from the same plant, a plant that yields a full spectrum of different colored teas with varying degrees of health benefits depending on said color. White, green, oolong, and black tea all come from the plant *Camellia sinensis.* In their rawest state, the tea leaves are green with white buds. As these are processed, the buds disappear, leaving only the green tea leaves; these are what give the tea its color. It is then fermented to oolong tea, a combination of green and black, and finally black tea.[4] You need to know the difference so you can understand why black tea and coffee lack health benefits and do nothing to alleviate physical or emotional stress.

White, oolong, and green tea all contain epigallocatechin gallates, or EGCGs, which are polyphenols.[7] Polyphenols are compounds that cause the body to expel more calories through heat. In green tea, they cause your body to burn approximately 4% more calories per day.[6] For someone burning 1,800 calories per day, this means that choosing a cup of green tea, rather than black tea or coffee, could help you burn as many as seventy more calories per day. If you drink a cup of green tea every day, that's over half a pound lost per month, or about seven pounds a year! The rawer the tea, the more polyphenols there are, and the more potential there is for fat loss through burning calories. In regard to tea production, this means that white tea burns more fat than green tea, green tea burns more fat than oolong tea, and oolong tea burns more fat than black tea. The same rule of thumb applies for health benefits like a tea's level of natural antioxidants. For this reason, choose white, green, and oolong tea over black tea.

On top of these health benefits, tea will still give you the kick you need to replace coffee. Specifically, green tea, oolong tea, white tea, and yerba maté tea contain caffeine and stimulants like caffeine. The difference is that these stimulants do not kick up as much adrenaline and noradrenaline as coffee. Understand that while adrenaline and noradrenaline do stimulate fat loss when excreted, too much is not a good thing since what goes up must come down. Basically, overstimulating adrenaline from using fat burners, black tea, or coffee will create more energy than you need to do simple mundane office work, dropping back down in a short time span, and robbing you of energy, drive, and focus when it does. This is bad enough for someone without diabetes, but diabetics will face a drop in blood sugar followed by subsequent carb cravings when it happens. This makes choosing tea over coffee for a pick-me-up even more attractive to our kind. The caffeine in green tea is surrounded by tannic acid, which causes the caffeine to be released more slowly than the caffeine found in coffee.[4] This means that the energizing effect happens gradually, lasts longer, and produces a less obvious crash than coffee.[4] Also recall these teas all contain theanine, that amino acid that keeps you calm. Since theanine actually works against overstimulation, the result is a more alert, less jittery focus that lasts longer, doesn't peak, and doesn't drop you. More specifically, yerba maté contains the methylxanthine maté, which is a stimulant much like caffeine. This particular stimulant, however, does not cause caffeine's nervous energy.[10] Because yerba maté has a tonic effect on the nervous system that calms the mind and body, it has also been found to promote sleep at the end of the day.

Teas can help you burn fat and lose weight. Even better, you'll be able to fall asleep at night if you're drinking two to four strong cups of tea rather than coffee. We diabetics can safely increase energy without overtaxing our system's reserves, ensuring our temporary solution to fatigue does not come with unwanted side effects of cravings, hunger, weight gain, and higher blood sugar. With these teas, you get pros without cons.

Using Amino Acids to Gain Control

You've already learned that stress depletes brain dopamine, the neurotransmitter responsible for attention, reward, motivation, and learning. The need for dopamine is the need to acquire more energy to do work, not to mention the subconscious belief that you will be rewarded for your efforts, thus motivating you to continue.

> **The top three ways people try to boost dopamine are through drinking coffee, smoking cigarettes, and eating heavy protein foods.**

Protein contains tyrosine, dopamine's building block, and fat and salt increase brain dopamine levels. Such combinations are found in pizza, Mexican and Italian cuisine, and cheeseburgers, cravings for which are subconscious attempts to increase dopamine. After eating them to regenerate from too much work, with internal compensation "earned," you find yourself with newfound energy to tackle the job at hand.

As you now understand, those food cravings and caffeine binges come with a price to diabetics. Even smoking is an extra burden on diabetics beyond the normal lung and heart risk since it's been shown to increase insulin resistance.[27] While nicotine increases both serotonin and dopamine levels and boosts energy, withdrawal from smoking drops serotonin and dopamine levels below normal, increasing moodiness and hunger.[21] So for a diabetic, smoking will make food cravings worse, which will make blood sugar control harder. In fact, abusing any of these methods while enduring other forms of stress chronically lowers dopamine. As a consequence, appetite for salt, protein, and fat goes through the roof[13] and the need for coffee or cigarettes perpetuates.[22]

A safer and natural alternative to all three types of dopamine cravings is to supplement your diet with amino acids. Just as you learned that taking 5-HTP increases serotonin in the brain, taking dopamine's building blocks accomplishes the analogous goal. So not surprisingly, taking 1,000 mg of L-tyrosine with 1,000 mg of L-phenylalanine twice a day on an empty stomach will give you the boost in drive and focus you would normally gain from coffee drinking.[11] Like tryptophan, these two amino acids are found in protein foods like meat, eggs, and dairy. Phenylalanine is used by the body to produce tyrosine, which you'll recall triggers dopamine, the brain's natural stimulant. In layman's terms, then, phenylalanine initiates a process that results in the brain becoming *naturally* stimulated. On top of that, phenylalanine also *counteracts* the symptoms of caffeine withdrawal[11] by keeping dopamine levels elevated, a job that caffeine had been doing for you until you quit. Tyrosine and phenylalanine supplementation will also help with nicotine withdrawals.[12]

> **While quitting regular coffee and smoking, you can take tyrosine for energy and phenylalanine to counter the withdrawals, avoiding excessive hunger and energy crashes. That makes**

these two amino acids a valuable tool for fighting insulin resistance, the true cause of high blood sugar in type II diabetics.

Tyrosine has several other beneficial side effects. To start, it's fantastic at helping you focus in the face of stress.[23-24] Really, you don't know that you're ever stressed. You know that you have lots of work you don't want to do plus no energy, and you *perceive* that as stress. That lack of motivation, focus, and energy is really dopamine going low from the body's stress. Tyrosine supplementation counters that. Likewise, if you find yourself wanting a big lunch, and you haven't recently expended enough calories to justify it, or you're working late and get pizza cravings, try 2,000 mg of both amino acids. Within half an hour, you'll be more focused, and beating those cravings. These amino acids are even great at combating the lethargic, unmotivated, can't-get-out-of-bed side of depression.[25-26] To understand why, you need to understand the two faces of clinical depression. One side is serotonin related – depression with low serotonin is the anxious, moody, carb-craving insomniac. These people respond well to SSRIs used to treat depression through raising brain serotonin. On the flip side, depression with low dopamine leaves you lifeless, exhausted, and unmotivated. You close the blinds, climb under the covers, and hide from the world. This form of depression is usually treated using a monoamine oxidase inhibitor (MAOI), a prescription drug specifically designed to increase dopamine in the brain. Not surprisingly then, supplementing with tyrosine helps.

You now understand that dopamine cravings can take the form of coffee, cigarette, and heavy protein cravings. Acting on any of these three is detrimental to your diabetes. All three will raise blood sugar and add to weight gain in one form or another. Further, they are only a temporary solution to your tired and stressed-out brain and body. For this reason, supplementing with tyrosine and phenylalanine is a more direct and natural way to treat the cause of your fatigue, low dopamine, without undesired side effects. You don't have to lose your mental edge at work. Better yet, you can keep it and your health at the same time.

- Cigarette smoking increases insulin resistance, so you should quit if you do smoke. Use tyrosine and phenylalanine alongside the patch as needed.
- While tyrosine does stimulate the adrenal glands and the thyroid like other stimulants, it does so to a lesser degree. For this reason, these natural stimulants are easily handled even by people who are caffeine sensitive.

Create a Stress Kit

You want to be prepared when stress hits because you can't always predict when it's going to happen. It's better to prevent a binge in the first place than try to exercise the results off. So go to an online site that sells supplements, like vitacost.com, and build a stress kit for yourself. Purchase the following:

1. One bottle of L-theanine tablets
2. One bottle of 5-HTP tablets
3. One bottle of L-glutamine in powder form
4. One bottle of L-tyrosine tablets
5. One box of Lipton or Celestial Seasonings' Caffeinated Green Tea.

Now build your stress kit. Put it in a nice box. Decorate it with inspiring notes to yourself, and the cards your daughter made you in her kindergarten class. Make it your best friend; something that makes you happy when you look at it. Keep it in a desk drawer at work, or wherever you encounter the most stress. You might find that you need one for work and another for home. But make sure you have it, and use it. This kit is your best friend, and your closest ally when it comes to dealing with stress. You should also print out the following instructions, so that you're prepared.

The next time you get exhausted, pull it out and take 1,000 to 2,000 mg of tyrosine with a strong cup of green tea. Be prepared to back that up with 50 to 200 mg of theanine one to three times per day. If you're experiencing sugar cravings take 2,000 mg of glutamine with 50 to 100 mg of 5-HTP. The strategy here is to control stress and energy by optimizing your hormones and neurotransmitters as safely as possible. This will help you prevent stress and emotional eating, which will go a long way in helping to maintain stable blood sugar. By avoiding potential pitfalls in your diet via simple strategies like taking amino acids at the right time, you can expect far better control over your diabetes year round. With or without using these supplements, remember that you are in control of what goes in your mouth, and therefore what your glucometer reads. However, taking these amino acids when needed will make it easier to make the right choice.

Continue to Support Your Body

Stress makes diabetes worse and researchers even debate whether stress is a direct cause of diabetes.

Either way, assisting the adrenal glands and immune system by providing them with the key nutrients to optimally function will go a long way in allowing the body to adapt to stress, which will go a long way in helping you control blood sugar. The adrenals need to be able to excrete cortisol and adrenaline as needed. Your body tissues need to receive those hormones without resistance. To that end, you'll want to take the following vitamins and minerals on a daily basis, to continue to give your body the support it needs. But don't bother if you aren't sleeping enough, or still abusing nicotine, caffeine, and alcohol.

Remove the negatives before you add positives.

Teas

As you've already read, white, green, oolong, and yerba maté teas are all superior to coffee and black tea in giving sustained energy and focus without adding on more stress by overtaxing the body. Unfortunately, not all brands of tea have the same concentration of polyphenols and methylxanthines, the active ingredients that make these teas potent energizers, stress fighters, and fat burners. You need 250 to 350 mg of polyphenols per day to get a fat-burning effect, which equates to three or four cups of a quality brand. Assays of many leading brands have shown that Lipton Green Tea and Celestial Seasonings Green Tea have the greatest number of polyphenols and EGCGs of all leading brands.[8-9] You'll probably have to visit an Asian market for white or oolong tea, or a green tea with a guaranteed high polyphenol count. Yerba maté is available at most health food stores and in some supermarkets.

Whether you have tea, coffee, or fat burners, they're all handled best by the body when taken with a meal. If you're going the tea route, you'll want to have one cup with each of your first three or four meals. If you're doing coffee, try one cup with breakfast, and a second in the afternoon, but no more.

Vitamins and Antioxidants[14]

Below are the most important nutrients that help the brain and body deal with stress. Most multivitamins will fall shy in one or more of these, but a high-quality-one will come pretty close. Just make sure you're sleeping more, eating better, and using less coffee before you start to worry whether you're getting enough magnesium in your life!

- Two to four grams of vitamin C
- 800 IU of vitamin E
- 1,500 mg of pantothenic acid
- 25 to 50 mg of niacin
- 50 to 100 mg of vitamin B_6
- 100 mg of vitamin B complex

- 250 to 500 mg of magnesium
- 750 to 1,000 mg of calcium
- 20 to 30 mg of zinc

Phosphatidyl Serine[15]

This supplement reduces cortisone levels. It's advised if you are under chronic stress. Take 300 to 800 mg in three divided dosages every day.

Herbs and extracts[14]

Licorice root, ashwagandha root, ginger root, adrenal cell extract are known as adaptogens, a term used to describe any and all compounds that help you adapt to stress, psychological or physical, anxiety, or fatigue. They are safe, and have been used for thousands of years in India and China. While they typically are only used to describe herbs, I list adrenal cell extracts here as well because it serves the same purpose as licorice, ashwagandha, and ginger – to help you cope better with stress. Adaptogens help your nervous system work more efficiently, allowing you to cope with stress easier. Since the dosage on each adaptogen varies, it's best to seek out an expert in herbal medicine to see if these will help.

Ginseng[14]

When it comes to supplements that help your body cope with stress, ginseng is at the top of the list. It increases energy, boosts the immune system, and lowers blood sugar. Specifically, it allows you to adapt to and cope with increased stress. Although either is OK, Siberian ginseng has a slight edge over Korean ginseng in aiding the body. Take one to two grams of high-quality crude Siberian or Korean ginseng three times a day, or 100 mg of standardized ginseng extract (5% ginsenosides) three times a day to alleviate stress and further boost energy.

Gingko Biloba[14]

Taking 120 to 160 mg of this herb increases blood flow to the brain, which enhances concentration. It also helps the adrenal glands to function properly. Shoot for brands of this herb that contain 24% of its active ingredient, flavonoid glycosides.

The Third Prescription in Summary

- Stress is a major cause of emotional eating.
- Lack of sleep is the number one stressor.
- 100 to 200 mg of L-theanine before bed can help you fall asleep, especially if caffeine or anxiety is keeping you awake.
- In general, it's best to limit caffeine intake to two cups of coffee, or 200 mg of caffeine per day from coffee. Too much caffeine impairs cognitive performance and adds to cravings.
- Theanine is responsible for the calming effect in green tea. Use it over coffee as a more moderate stimulant. It also helps you burn more fat and calories.
- If you regularly suffer from insomnia, wake up recurrently during the night, or have trouble getting into a deep sleep, have 1-3 mg of melatonin with 200 to 400 mg of 5-HTP one hour before bedtime.
- 1,000 to 2,000 mg of both L-tyrosine and L-phenylalanine can help with energy, focus, quitting coffee and cigarettes, and eliminating cravings for fat, protein, and salt.

Moving On with Your Life

The litmus test to knowing you're no longer a stress eater is if you can *eat the same foods in the same quantities nine times out of ten come hell or high water no matter what has happened to you that day or week.* The solutions you learn throughout this book will begin your journey to learn how to do just that.

FOURTH PRESCRIPTION

Exercise Is the Best Medication

The purpose of diabetes medication is to lower blood sugar. Unfortunately, that sometimes comes with side effects like weight gain since a lot of the meds work by increasing total insulin, our greatest fat-storage hormone (the meds that strictly help the body use insulin better cause weight loss as you'll learn in the coming chapter). Contrast that knowledge with the fact that weight loss is bar none the greatest "cure" for type II diabetes. Wouldn't it be nice to have a method that lowers blood sugar, helps the body use insulin better and need less of it, and causes weight loss? We do, available without prescription or copay! It's called exercise! When done right, it really can be as effective as medication. Let me tell you a story.

I used to lift weights with my friend Eric, a fellow diabetic, who is also a doctor. During our workouts, and for hours after, we'd check our blood sugar religiously. Why? Using our glucometers, we confirmed our symptoms of dizziness, confusion, and hunger were caused by very low blood sugar. I had blood sugar readings as low as 40 mg/dl as long as twenty-four hours after exercise.

Exercise is really effective at lowering blood sugar!

Exercise doesn't stop working when you stop moving. It's like a pill. It works for the whole day.

Eric is a wonderful example of the power that exercise has to control blood sugar. He is an insulin-dependent diabetic from his battle with cystic fibrosis, a disease that can cause diabetes in over 50% of its adult population. The majority of diabetics with insulin-dependent diabetes mellitus (IDDM) are type I diabetic (accounting for 10% of all diabetics), caused by an autoimmune disease where the body destroys the islets of Langerhans, where the cells that manufacture insulin in the pancreas are located. Like all those with IDDM, Eric's pancreas produces barely any insulin, meaning he has to inject insulin to survive. But exercise has drastically reduced how much insulin Eric needs to take. At his most active, he has used one-third of the normal amount of insulin for a man of his size. So even if you must take insulin, exercise can reduce the amount you need.

Likewise, exercise is 50% of the reason I'm not on insulin right now. The other 50% is how I eat. Think about that. One hour of effort is half of the reason I don't use insulin, while twenty-three hours of eating well makes up the other half. That's one powerful hour!

Studies show that exercise will lower blood sugar in every diabetic just like it has for me and Eric. A study done at a Pritikin Longevity Center in conjunction with UCLA found that 71% of noninsulin-dependent diabetics who exercised intensely each day were able to stop taking their oral medications after three weeks, and another 39% stopped using insulin (taking insulin for them was a choice, not a necessity)! The same study found 34% of the subjects on blood pressure medication were able to completely stop taking them. The average subject also cut their bad cholesterol 22%, and triglycerides 33%[18]. You need multiple medications to achieve such control in all three of these facets of diabetes, drugs that can drain your energy and pocketbook while leaving you overweight, albeit with better blood sugar, blood pressure, and cholesterol than if you'd done nothing at all.

That medication solution will help your diabetes, but at the cost of keeping you heavier than if you chose to control it with exercise. All diabetes medications that cause weight gain rob you of the ability to control the disease through weight loss. Exercise doesn't do that. That's why it's a better long-term solution. If you still need prescriptions to control diabetes after having exercised intensely for a while, you'll get by on ones that don't cause weight gain, making the disease much more manageable long term.

The pills aren't magic. You are capable of being just as effective as a doctor in controlling type II diabetes. Further, consider that Januvia, Metformin, Byetta, Precose, and Glyset are the only type II drugs out of about twenty that *don't* cause weight gain. They work either to increase the effectiveness of the insulin you do have, or to slow the rate or total amount of glucose entering the blood. What they don't do is get your body to increase the total amount of insulin, which is why these drugs don't cause weight gain (much more on medications is found in the Ninth Prescription, titled Know Your Diabetic Complications, Their Medications, and Your Alternatives). So if you're trying to lose weight, and taking a medication that causes weight gain, you're obviously going to have a harder time.

Even if you're happy on the prescriptions you're taking now, medical statistics show that medications for diabetes become less and less effective after about five years, meaning you'll need to go on more powerful pills. Over time, diabetes gets worse in all of us, but the medication dosage remains the same. Even if this wasn't happening, the drugs that cause the pancreas to excrete more insulin may exhaust the organ over time, leading to less and less insulin excretion, and higher and higher blood sugar. If you don't exercise, you'll need more meds or higher dosages of the ones you're already on to maintain control. Weight gain will be a guarantee well before that time since diabetic control will be falling. All of a sudden, forty-five minutes of exercise doesn't sound *so bad*...

Exercise Lessens the Amount of Insulin Needed

Exercise improves blood sugar not only by inducing fat loss, but by lowering the amount of insulin needed by the body to process nutrients. However, not all exercise is equal in these abilities. Walking is better than nothing, but it's nothing compared to weight lifting. Lifting weights increases muscle, which permanently lowers insulin resistance. Muscle tissue is very metabolically active and needs a lot of nutrients to thrive, making it very receptive to glucose.

> **While all forms of exercise help transfer glucose into your cells *independent* of insulin,[1] intense forms do it best.[2] Intense exercise causes the diabetic body to work as efficiently as it would if insulin was fully present and active.**

Insulin is the body's primary transporter of glucose. The secondary transportation system is commonly known as GLUT, an acronym for "glucose transporter." The harder or longer the exercise, and the more muscle built, the harder GLUT will work for the body. Since GLUT needs exercise and muscle to happen, the more muscle or more intense the exercise, the more GLUT. So long as you exercise and maintain your muscle, GLUT is working for you. Incredibly, nothing else in nature is known to do this. That's how Eric was able to cut his injectable insulin usage so dramatically. This gives you a very simple way to control insulin and blood sugar *without* having to resort to a pill or needle. And you get the added benefit of health and weight loss. Weight lifting will also do wonders for your cholesterol and blood pressure.[3] It really is the ultimate prescription, which is why it's fourth on your list.

Again, this is something that's been backed by scientific study. When twenty-six men with type II diabetes or prediabetes engaged in a twenty-week exercise program, utilizing either cardiovascular or strength-training exercise, those who exercised significantly decreased their serum glucose and insulin levels by the end of the study.[4] The control group who didn't exercise did not. This study differs from the one previously mentioned in that this one had a control that proves not exercising does not improve blood sugar.

> **The magic of this concept is that exercise will begin lowering your blood sugar and promoting a healthy body immediately, no matter how long it's been since you last exercised.**

After researchers tested sedentary middle-aged men who exercised for fourteen weeks, both their glucose transporters and insulin sensitivity just about doubled.[5] These were men who had been inactive up to that point, seeing results in a little over three months. And these were impressive results, especially in regard to what they could mean for a typical diabetic. When insulin sensitivity doubles, it means that it takes half the amount of insulin to move a given amount of glucose into cells. That kind of natural effect drastically cuts into the amount of medication a diabetic might need. This makes exercise the greatest natural "cure" for type II diabetes. It literally reverses insulin resistance and simultaneously provides an alternative way to transport glucose without even needing insulin, even if you're just starting out.

The lesson here is very important. Don't think that you can just eat differently to control your weight and blood sugar. Your ancestors lived much more actively than you do, and type II diabetics was nonexistent, for a very good reason. They were more physically active. Exercise can be the answer to controlling your diabetes. I told you I would not ask you for much of your time. But I will ask for your dedication and consistency with the time you give.

That means that it doesn't matter how busy your job or family life is. I can even find the time to exercise with a six-year-old boy running around me. We have lightsaber battles between sets. Even most presidents exercise every day.[6] And the presidency has been described as the most stressful job in the world. What responsibilities do you have that are greater? There are ER doctors working eighty-hour weeks who find the time. You have no excuses. So if you're ready to make that commitment, move into this Prescription.

Three Questions You Must Answer to Set Up Your Program

One size does not fit all when it comes to exercise. Squats may help your friend, but maybe you have hip arthritis. Running might be fine for your spouse, but maybe you've recently suffered a heart attack. Two-hour bouts at the gym three days a week might work better for your neighbor, but maybe you can only devote forty minutes a day. That's why before you begin, you need to answer these questions.

1. How much time are you willing and able to commit to exercise every week? It doesn't have to be the same amount every day, but it should total about 300 minutes for the week.

2. What physical restrictions do you have? Do you have any injuries or health conditions that make some forms of exercise impossible?

3. What is the deep-seated reason that you are going to commit to doing this day in and day out for the rest of your life? It can't be spousal revenge, and it can't be a high school reunion. What's going to get you up at 6 AM, after only five hours of sleep, to work out? What's going to make you find the time while you're on vacation? What's going to make you find the time while you're on a business trip? You now know that the general benefits of exercise are increased energy and disease prevention, along

with the usual physical improvements, but what do those attributes mean in your life? What benefits do they pose to you? How do they make you feel? Are those reasons strong enough to overcome schedule restraints and lack of sleep? If they are, you've found your answer. If they aren't, keep looking, because the answers do lie inside you.

We'll deal with your answer to the first question by breaking up the exercise program featured below into time frames that you can do. It's quite simple. Later, as you learn to develop your own exercise programs, you'll naturally understand how much exercise per day accommodates your goals and lifestyle. For now, break the program given in this chapter into the time you have.

The exercise program itself has been designed to be friendly on the joints, but if you experience discomfort or have a preexisting injury, you should consult an orthopedic specialist for any modifications you may need. Your doctor *must* go over your physical limitations with you to help you decide which types of exercise are right for you and which might cause injury. Exercise is safe, but only as safe as you are smart. Be smart, and get clearance from your doctor before you start, regardless of whether you have obvious limits or not. You can also contact me at my website, http://www.TheNew-DiabetesPrescription.com, for more help.

The third question's answer is the most important. You will inevitably stop exercising unless it becomes a part of your soul. You must find a love for it. It may not happen at first (and often it won't), but it must happen. The only way you will find that intrinsic impulse is if you start doing it. I know how hard it can be to start. And I speak from experience. From age five to about eleven, I was stuck in special education PE with all the physically and mentally challenged kids because I was so inactive. I couldn't throw a ball, and I didn't even know the basic rules of any sport. I spent my days indoors, playing with Legos. I saw nothing wrong with this kind of lifestyle, but my parents and school had different ideas. I complemented this inactive lifestyle with lots of junk food, eating fast food for dinner nearly five nights a week. I'm certain this accelerated the onset of my diabetes by decades.

My lifelong affair with exercise began the day my best friend in the eighth grade fell in love with a girl who was joining the high school cross-country team. He joined to be close to her, and my other best friend wanted to have the same PE class, so he joined as well. I didn't want to be left behind, so I did the same. Only then did I ask what exactly cross-country was.

As it turned out, my high school had the top cross-country team in the country. It was led by a coach so dedicated to running that he had actually lost his arm after being bitten by a rattlesnake during a race. He was in the lead, ran into some brush where the snake was hiding, got bit. The closest medical aid was at the finish line, so he decided to finish the race, but his rapid heart rate from running accelerated the poison through his arm, and the doctors had to amputate it to save his life. The "one-armed pirate," as he came to be known, pushed us week after week. We ran two miles the first day, and I had to walk the last half. For the first month, I offered to pay people to walk with me so I wouldn't be the only one. I spent the entire season finishing last or close to last in every race. It was embarrassing, and it was hard.

Interestingly, I never noticed that week by week I was able to run longer distances. Every week the coach added a mile to the running assignments, and I mindlessly obeyed. I was actually getting in better shape without realizing it. What I did notice was the fatigue, pain, and embarrassment. I was miserable, but I refused to quit. I'd walk the distance if I had to, but I'd never drop out. And then one night everything changed. We were required to run on the weekends for practice, and I was running on my own. The air was perfect, and my energy was high. I ran five miles so easily that it felt like I was gliding. I was actually enjoying myself, for the first time. And I remember that five miles better than the 1,000 negative experiences that led up to it. It didn't matter how many times I had been out of breath or suffering from shin splints; the difference I felt in that one positive run had me hooked. From then on, I sought to duplicate that feeling of ultimate joy and power every time I exercised. It became something I anticipated and even craved. So this is how I came to love exercise. It's my answer to question 3.

Am I a saint? Do I have some indomitable soul that can endure bludgeoning after bludgeoning until I finally reach the Promised Land? Not at all: it's actually simpler than that. Physical activity is a part of being human, and it's part of being alive. Our bodies are built to move. You're not truly living life if you're not using your body the way it was meant to be used. And it makes sense that something so fundamental to survival would feel good. Why does fear of famine or being killed or losing a loved one have to be the only emotions that drive one to action? Why can't positive emotions do the same? They can, and that is why I exercise.

So why will you?

1. How much time are you willing and able to commit to exercise every week?
2. What physical restrictions do you have?
3. What is the deep-seated reason that you are going to commit to doing this day in and day out for the rest of your life?

Stop reading until you've answered all three questions, and write down your answers where you can see them. Now that you have them, you'll need to learn one more step before you can dive into The New Diabetes Exercise Prescription – injury prevention.

Injury Prevention Is the Key to Success

I'll bet you can name at least one person who was over-exuberant in trying to whip themselves into shape, only to wind up injured. Maybe they hurt their back, their knee, or their shoulder. Even if you don't know someone to whom this happened, I'll bet you or someone you know has a nagging pain that just won't go away. In either case, trigger points, little knots in your muscles, were a contributor.

Trigger points arise from a variety of sources, and a diabetic is guaranteed to have more than average since inactivity and nutritional deficiencies are both major causes. They manifest themselves as sharp, burning, or diffuse pain at the location of the trigger point, or even far away. For example, a trigger point in the upper part of your butt, the gluteus minimus, can manifest itself as classic sciatica, pain running down your leg all the way to your toes. Releasing the knot in your butt makes the pain in your leg go away!

Trigger points do more than cause pain. When a muscle has a knot, it doesn't produce force as well (which is the purpose of muscle), meaning its synergists, muscles that help the particular muscle's function, must pick up the slack, leading to overuse and injury. Similarly, a tight muscle means that particular muscle's opposite or agonist does not fire as well. For example, having tight hip flexors means your glute muscles cannot extend as well, meaning your lower back and hamstrings have to pick up the slack, causing back strains and hamstring pulls. This is a common problem that can be solved if you know how to get rid of the knot.

Because it's a knot, stretching a trigger point does not make it go away, and can often make it worse. If you have a knot in a rope, and pull it tighter, the knot becomes harder to untangle. This analogy is perfect because muscles are fibers, and trigger points are knots in those fibers. Stretch a muscle by pulling on those fibers, and you tighten the knot. The solution is to perform a type of massage known as myofascial self-release, which roughly translates to "get rid of those knots yourself!"

A list of all the trigger points in the body and how they manifest is beyond the scope of this book. But getting rid of 90% of them with one tool and one technique is not. You will therefore use a foam roller on your muscles prior to even warming up to ensure you have no knots in your body.

A foam roller is a roll of hard foam, six to eight inches in diameter, that you can buy from most sporting goods stores. Considering it will cost you between $10 and $15, it is the second cheapest massage tool you'll ever get. The cheapest, a simple tennis ball, costs a tenth as much as a foam roller, but hurts ten times more. It's a good investment six months from now when most of your trigger points are under control, but it's too painful right now. Regardless, any knot, tightness, or pain that is muscular in origin can be relieved by lying on the floor on top of the roller, and rolling the afflicted area up and down on the roller for six to twelve times. Perform the below sequence at least once before exercising, or any time you are in pain.

The New Diabetes Trigger Point Therapy

Here are some tips for getting the most out of this basic piece of equipment:

- Use your foam roller on any muscle that is tight before you start exercising.
- When rolling very slowly up and down the muscle, the more pressure you can put on the area the better. Roll where it hurts, keep on it for thirty seconds, and then keep rolling down away from the painful area.
- The muscle you're trying to roll should be on top of the foam ruler, i.e., perpendicular to it.
- You may use a medicine ball in place of a foam roller now, and a tennis ball months from now.
- Once you've finished rolling, it is then an appropriate and optimal time to stretch, as the knots have been released, and stretching will keep them away. Hold the stretches at the end of this section for thirty seconds each.
- If you feel absolutely nothing in the muscles because you have a lot of fat in the area you're trying to roll, you may omit the exercise for now. As you firm up, try again. Once you feel the massage actually taking place on the muscle, you'll want to stick with it!

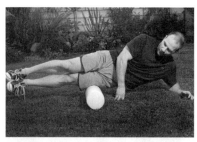

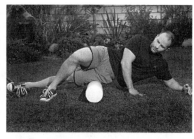

Rolling the Lower Side of the Leg

Rolling the Upper Side of the Leg

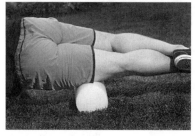

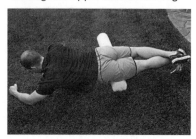

Rolling the Lower Front
Part of the Thigh

Rolling the Upper Front
Part of the Thigh

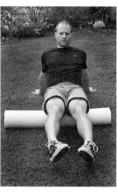

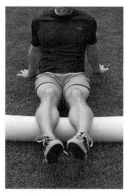

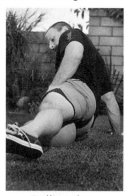

Rolling the
Hamstrings

Rolling the Calves

Rolling the
Peroneus

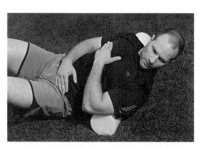

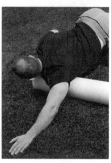

Rolling the Lats and Upper Back

Rolling the Pecs

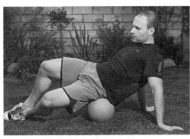
Rolling the Glutes

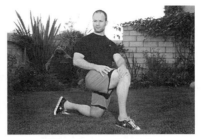
Hip Flexors Stretch

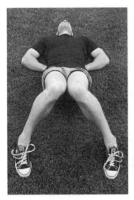
Internal Rotators
Stretch

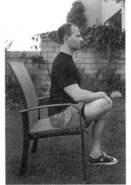
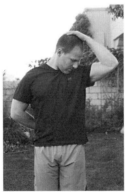
External Rotators Stretch
Note that my lower back does not round

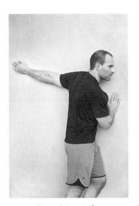
Pec Stretch   Levator Scapulae Stretch

113

Exercise Is the Best Medicine

How to Start Working Out

The best exercise to get you into shape comes in three flavors:

- Low-intensity aerobic exercise.
- Weight lifting, a form of anaerobic exercise.
- High-intensity aerobic exercise, which is in truth anaerobic exercise with spurts of aerobic exercise mixed between.

You're going to perform all three forms in this order. As you'll learn below, there are important advantages and disadvantages to each, and important guidelines for how and how *not* to do each one. We'll start by learning a little more about aerobic exercise in general, and then learn the New Diabetes Aerobic Program.

Cardiovascular Exercise Is a Great Place to Start

Cardiovascular exercise trains the heart, lungs, and blood vessels to more efficiently pump oxygenated blood throughout the body.

It decreases the resting heart rate and increases the body's oxygen consumption. Like all forms of exercise, it can lower blood pressure, cholesterol, and blood sugar while burning fat. Depending on how many beats per minute your heart is going, it can be divided roughly into low, medium, and high intensity. We'll start with the easiest kind that everyone can do, and progress from there.

Low-intensity cardiovascular exercise is loosely classified as any movement you can perform for at least twenty minutes while carrying on a conversation. That leaves a lot of wiggle room. Walking, dancing, running, skiing, swimming, hiking, rock climbing, and a thousand other activities all fall under this definition, depending on your current fitness level. These activities are a lot of fun, very social, and can burn a lot of calories, especially if you're doing something like running, swimming, or using an exercise machine at the gym. For anyone out of shape or just starting to exercise, a brisk walk can also qualify as low-intensity cardio. These are all great ways to start whipping your body into shape. They're also great to be included as a warm-up to more strenuous exercise since they get the blood flowing and raise core body temperature. This prepares the body to exert itself with less chance of injury.

Disadvantages to low-intensity cardio are few and far between, but the truth is that there are better ways to lose weight and control diabetes. For example, walking will take at least three times longer than jogging to burn the same number of calories. What's more, the calorie-burning effect from walking stops as soon as the walking stops. This isn't the case with high-intensity forms of exercise like running, interval training, or weight lifting. These more intense forms of exercise leave your metabolism elevated for as long as forty-eight hours after you're done! This means that you actually burn more calories in the days following hard exercise than you do while doing it. When low-intensity exercise is over, so are the benefits. To put it another way, walking (low-intensity) is like collecting a paycheck by working forty-hour weeks, while weight lifting (high-intensity) is like collecting rent checks from an apartment building that you own. How would you rather earn your income (burn your calories)? Think of weight lifting as investment property. Once you put in the money (physical effort), you reap the rewards (fat loss). And fat loss is the number one solution for type II diabetes. If it wasn't, doctors would not be encouraging stomach stapling!

More intense forms of exercise result in more fat loss in less time.

So given that low-intensity cardio is great for beginners and great for warming up, I've created a traditional warm-up program of body-weight-only exercises that you can move through several times, giving you the following advantages:

1. It will burn calories, and it can be the only low-intensity cardio you ever need to do except walking, which is inevitable.

2. It's built from dynamic mobility drills, exercises that are like stretches held for less than two seconds at a time, shown to prepare the muscles, joints, tendons, and nervous system for weight lifting. Stretching does not do this since stretching is done to lengthen muscles, and not mobilize joints – that is the major difference.

3. It will improve posture by lengthening tight muscles and strengthening weak ones while acting as an aerobic program that tones the body.

4. It will get you out of pain. Living with diabetes can hurt. The hormonal and nutritional deficiencies and excess weight caused by diabetes predisposes you to backaches, disc issues, muscle cramps and tightness, and frozen shoulders. Sitting at a desk for half your life only exacerbates these imbalances, locking in pain and locking you out of the body you want. The routine below will improve your mobility to start alleviate those old pains.

Follow the One-Hour Rule

Move for one hour every day, or 300 minutes per week. Just pick yourself up, put on your iPod, and go. If you finish your weight lifting workout with fifteen minutes to spare, do something else for another fifteen. Just move for that one hour. It can be any form of exercise you can and will do. If you have access to an exercise machine like a stationary bike, and you prefer that to walking, that is fine. *But* try to go a little harder in the given amount of time as the weeks go by. Also, if you want to exercise for thirty minutes in the morning, and another thirty at night, that's fine. Again, just move for that one hour. And longer is fine when you have the time.

Move for one hour every day.

The New Diabetes Aerobic Program

Besides doing these drills as cardio, you will also go through this entire sequence once or twice before every weight-training session. You will perform these exercises in the exact order provided, in a circuit fashion. So if you're only doing the sequence once, that's one circuit. If you move through the whole program twice, that's two circuits, and so on. Once you're good at it, moving through a single circuit should take eight to ten minutes. So when doing these movements for cardio, perform three to five circuits for a twenty-five-to fifty-minute workout. Perform eight to ten repetitions of each exercise in the program.

If you would prefer to do some other form of low-intensity exercise in addition to or instead of this routine below, you still must go through the entire circuit once or twice prior to lifting weights, no exceptions.

The first time you move through the program, I would recommend performing only two circuits if you find it difficult. Strive to add a circuit until you can do four or five without rest. In fact, you'll know you're ready for more intense cardiovascular exercise when you can do that without needing to stop to catch your breath.

Note: Where it reads to alternate arms or legs with each repetition, that means do one for the left, then one for the right, and so on until you've done ten to twelve reps for each side.

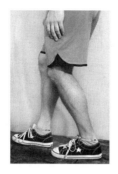

Ankle Mobilizations. This exercise mobilizes the ankle joint, which will take stress off your knees, hips, and lower back. While holding on to a wall or any other unmovable object, move your right foot forward and lock it into place. Now, rock your left leg forward as in the picture, ensuring that your heel remains on the floor at all times. You should feel your ankles becoming more and more mobile with each repetition. Do all reps for one leg before switching to the other.

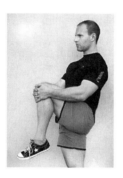

Knee Up. This exercise improves hip mobility to help you move from your hips instead of your lower back. While standing, pull your knee as close to your chest as possible, keeping your lower back arched, not rounded, ramrod straight the entire time. At the same time, flex your calf muscles on the opposite leg so that you're on your toes. Alternate legs.

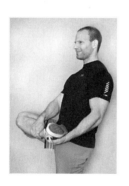

Cradle Walk. This exercise mobilizes the glutes and piriformis muscle, again helping with hip mobility. Pull your right leg at the ankle up and over to the opposite side of your body as shown in the picture. Simultaneously get up on your toes with the left leg. Maintain that arch in your lower back. You should feel a nice stretch in the hips. Move back and forth between legs for each rep. If necessary, you can lean against a wall the first few times for balance.

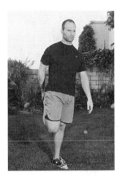

Butt Kick. This exercise mobilizes the quadriceps. Pull your leg up behind you until the back of your ankle touches your butt as shown in the photo. Simultaneously, get onto your toes with the opposite leg. As you do, be sure that the leg you're holding behind you is not going out to the side. Strive to keep your other leg right under your body. Hold on to a wall or solid object for support if needed. Alternate legs with each repetition.

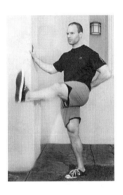

Leg Swing. This exercise increases hamstring mobility. Stand beside a wall and hold a hand against it for balance. Swing your leg rapidly back and forth, going as far forward and as far backward as possible. Make sure only your leg, and not your torso, is moving. You should feel this in the front of your hip and in your hamstrings. My hand is on the small of my lower back to ensure that I don't round my lower back as my leg moves forward. Do all reps for one leg before switching to the other.

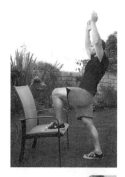

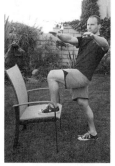

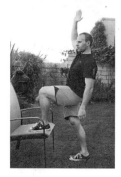

3-D Lunges. Lunges loosen the hip flexors so that the glutes can function better, taking stress off your lower back. Place your foot on a chair or stool as shown, with arms down at your sides, and the foot of your trailing leg facing straight ahead. Hold this position for the next three motions. As shown in the first photo on the left, lift both arms overhead as high as possible, trying to put them behind your body. You should feel an intense stretch in the back leg's hip flexor, where the front of your leg attaches to your pelvis. Do eight to ten reps and then position both arms straight out in front of you, parallel to the ground, palms facing down. As shown in the second photo in the middle, rotate *from your hips, not your lower back,* toward the leg on the stool. *You'll know you're doing it right if you feel the stretch in the same area, and not your lower back.* It helps on all of these to have your torso slightly leaning back as shown in the photos. Do eight to ten reps, and then raise the arm in the air opposite to the one on the stool as shown in the third photo. This time kick your hips out in the direction of the leg that is on the ground on each repetition. Again you should feel a stretch in the back leg's hip flexor, and to the side of it. Do all reps for this leg, then switch legs, and repeat all three exercises for the other side.

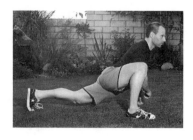

Spider Man. This is a great exercise for the inner thighs and hip flexors. Get into position by lunging forward with your right leg. Steadying yourself with your left hand firmly on the ground, with your right elbow, push your right leg outward as shown in the picture. You should feel a nice stretch in the inner thigh of your right leg. From here, while maintaining this posture, bring your right elbow away from your right leg and back on each repetition. Essentially, you're quickly mobilizing your front leg's inner thigh by pushing that thigh outward with your elbow, and then releasing the tension by taking your elbow out of contact with that leg. Do all reps for one leg before switching to the other.

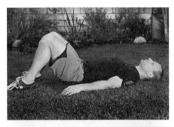
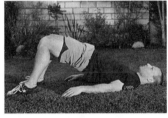

Glute Bridge. This exercise engages the glutes, which become dormant from too much sitting, adding to back pain. Lie on your back with your feet flat on the ground and your knees bent as shown on the photo on the left. Place your arms on the ground along your body, and keep them there. Squeeze your gluteal muscles (butt) to lift your torso as high off the ground as possible, but don't overarch your back. Keep pushing up, but stop before you feel the tension in your lower back instead of your glutes. This is a butt exercise!

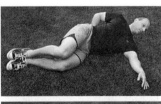
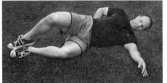

C-Clam. This exercise is extremely effective at working the gluteus medius at the side of your hips. Begin by lying on your left side, your left hand out in front of you, your legs together, and knees bent at ninety degrees. Your legs themselves should be flexed forty to sixty degrees forward of your pelvis, and your other hand is gently bracing the small of your back to remind you not to round there. You may place a pillow or small object beneath your head for more comfort. Holding this position, extend your top leg by flexing the upper hip. You should feel a contraction on the side of the hip that's facing upward, known as your gluteus medius. Lower and repeat. Do all reps for one leg before switching to the other.

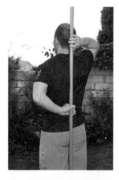

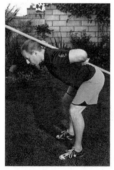

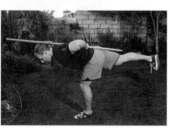

Two-Legged & One-Legged Deadlifts (Broom Handle Deadlifts). Besides mobilizing the hips and hamstrings, this exercise teaches you to use your butt instead of your lower back to pick things up. Get a broom handle or long light rod, and position it behind you as shown on the left. Ensure that the rod is firmly touching the back of your head, between your shoulder blades, and your butt. Your lower hand is between the rod and the small of your back. Your upper hand is between the rod and your neck. Do not let the rod leave contact with these three positions at any time during the exercises. Your feet may be slightly pointed outward as shown. You are now going to learn to hinge from the hips instead of the lower back. Bend forward by *pushing your hips back further and further*. Notice that if you try to bend from the waist, your back tries to round and the rod breaks contact with one of the three points. Instead, fold forward by pushing the hips back. You'll naturally notice that you're able to hold the rod in place and get deeper and deeper. Do eight to ten repetitions, and then get on one leg as shown in the last photo. Initiate hinging forward by *pushing the back leg back*. You are not initially expected to get down as far as I do in the photo, and you will find balancing this movement hard at first. But it will get easier with practice. Switch the hand positions, and repeat both movements again from the other side of the body.

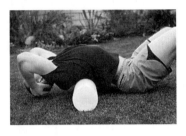

Thoracic Extensions. This exercise mobilizes your middle back so you can arch from there, taking stress off your lower back, neck, and shoulders. Lie on the floor with your feet flat on the floor and your knees bent. Place your foam roller across your middle back. Grasp the back of your head as shown in the photo, striving to keep your elbows pointing straight up through the movement. With your butt firmly on the ground, begin to extend the spine back as far as you can comfortably go, and come back. You can also try to do this a little higher or lower, but don't perform this on your lower back or neck. You can also use a medicine ball or two tennis balls taped together with athletic tape for this exercise.

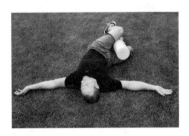

Thoracic Rotations. It's not enough to be able to extend the middle back. You must regain your ability to rotate from there to reap the benefits of less shoulder and back pain. Lie sideways on the ground with the foam roller between your knees as shown. Begin with your legs bent at right angles both at the hips and knees, and top arm lying over your bottom arm. Slowly extend the top arm all the way back until it is touching the ground behind you as shown in the picture. Bring the arm back, and repeat. Do all reps for one side before switching to the other.

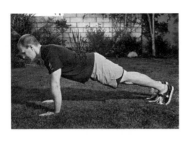

Push-Ups. Push-ups work the serratus muscle to keep the shoulders healthy. Do push-ups, keeping your upper arms as close to your body as possible. As you go down, your arms should remain close to your body. You can make the push-ups harder by putting your feet on a stool and bringing your hands closer together. You can also make them easier by pushing up from your knees instead of your toes.

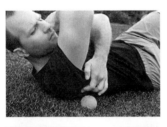

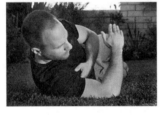

Subscapular Rotations. The subscapularis muscle is a common site of pain and restriction for the shoulder joint. This exercise will change that. Bring your arm across your shoulder while lying on one side, and find the bony protrusion just beneath your armpit. I'm pointing to it in the picture above on the left. Place the tennis ball there as shown in the first photo. From here, begin to do a series of rotations, externally rotating the arm all the way to the ground away from your head, and internally rotating it back to the ground toward your feet. You will know the right area because it will hurt like a good massage. Apply as much pressure as you can tolerate. Do all reps for one side before switching to the other.

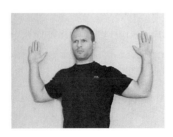

Wall Slides. This exercise activates the lower trapezius between the shoulder blades to keep the shoulder joint injury free. The photo shows the bottom of the movement. Stand against a wall in the position shown with your feet, butt, upper back, arms, and back of your head all touching the wall. While keeping all of these body parts tensed against the wall at all times, extend your hands as high as possible, reaching the classic "hands up" position. Ensure your forearms and elbows are still touching the wall at the very top. You should feel the muscles in your upper back contracting hard here. Now slide your arms back down along the wall as low as possible, as if trying to make your upper arms touch the sides of your body as shown in the photo.

The New Diabetes Weight Lifting Program

Go to your local sporting goods store and buy the following:

1. A pair of ten, fifteen, and twenty pound dumbbells if you're female, or a pair of fifteen, twenty-five, and thirty-five pound dumbbells if you're male.

2. Three exercise bands and three exercise cords of different resistance. Resistance bands are basically tough rubber loops. Resistance cords are the same concept, usually made from different materials, and are open-ended. They are widely available in most sporting goods stores, gym warehouses, and online.

3. A stopwatch.

4. Optional but highly recommended: a kettlebell found at a gym warehouse or online (12 kg for women, and 16 kg for men). These are now even available at Target. If you don't buy the kettlebell, you then must purchase two ten-pound weight plates if female, and a thirty-five pound weight plate if male. But a kettlebell is preferable.

5. A foam roller.

This is all the equipment you need for your home workouts. The total cost will be less than $100. The cost savings over your lifetime will be immeasurable considering the health benefits they'll give you.

Organizing Your Program

1. How Often Should You Work Out: The program below should be performed three times per week on nonconsecutive days (e.g., Monday, Wednesday, Friday or Friday, Sunday, Tuesday).

2. In What Order Should the Exercise Be Done: These twelve exercises should be done in the order given, which amounts to one circuit. To ease into exercising and cut down on soreness, perform only one circuit the first two times you do the program and two circuits the second two times you do the program. From then onward, stick with three circuits.

3. How Do You Know Which Weight Is Right for You: Select a weight where you could do one more rep than the number recommended (e.g., a weight you could eleven times if you're told to do ten). It is OK to not get it right the first time, going heavier or lighter than required. The correct weight will eventually become apparent.

4. The Importance of Proper Form: Proper exercise form is more important than anything else. Maintain good posture, don't jerk the weights, don't lift super slow, and in truth, try to lift the weights as quickly as possible with good form, and lower them under control. This will maximize the muscle-gain and fat-loss effects.

5. How Long Between Exercises: Have the stopwatch strapped to your wrist. As soon as you finish the set, make sure you get to the next one in a minute or less.

6. Keep Moving to Keep the Exercising Effective: Walk between sets! Don't sit down!

7. Increasing the Effectiveness of Your Workout: Fat loss here is achieved as you get through these circuits in less and less time. You do want to get stronger and do the exercises with heavier and heavier weight, but not at the expense of needing to rest more. For this reason, your

goal is to be able to get through each circuit resting less than thirty seconds between sets. Once you achieve that, increase the weight to where you need sixty seconds of rest between sets again. Then your goal will be to again get the rest time back down to thirty seconds with the heavier weight. Continue this process, adding weight, getting the rest time down under thirty seconds, and then adding weight again.

8. The Cool-Down Process: You may want to stretch at the end of your workout. Typically, you can hold stretches for thirty to forty-five seconds at a time. Use the ones outlined at the end of the New Diabetes Trigger Point Therapy section. If something else is tight that is not hit by those stretches, you can turn the cardio drills you learned in the New Diabetes Prescription Aerobics Program into stretches by holding them longer. For example, to stretch your inner thighs, hold the Spider Man for thirty to forty-five seconds. To stretch your quads, hold the Butt Kick for thirty to forty-five seconds, and so on.

The New Diabetes Prescription Exercises

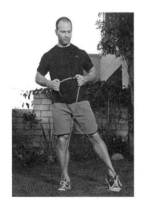

1) Mini-Band Side Steps (glutes). Grasp a band with both hands, stand on it, and then twist it so it makes an "X" as shown in the picture. Keeping your body rigid and your legs locked, "walk" sideways by moving your right leg to the side, followed by your left leg. Repeat until you've walked the desired number of steps to the right. Repeat these steps, moving toward the left. You should feel your hips contracting during this exercise. Do ten reps per side.

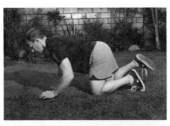

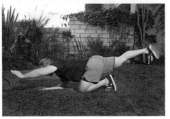

2) Super Bird Dogs (abdominals and lower back). Get on hands and knees, with your back arched. Extend your left arm straight out, while extending your right leg straight back. Your right arm and left leg will still be on the ground while the left arm and right leg are pointing outward, parallel to the ground. In the second photo, you'll see my left leg is significantly flexed, where the back of my leg almost touches my heel, and my torso is angled slightly downward. This is what makes it super – the deviation engages the glutes more. Hold this "bird dog" position for five seconds, and reverse sides. One hold on both sides counts as one rep. Do five reps per side.

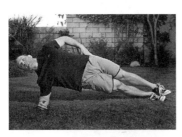

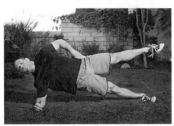

3) Side Bridges (obliques, and lower back). Lie on your right side, supporting yourself with your right elbow and foot (these should be the only parts of your body touching the ground). Your left leg should be balanced on top of your right leg, with your torso hiked toward the sky, and your pelvis in line with your chest. Ideally, your entire body should be straight, with absolutely no drooping of your body toward the ground. If this is too difficult, bend your legs ninety degrees. Or, to make it harder, keep the top leg elevated for the entire movement as shown in the second photo. Alternate sides, holding the pose for ten seconds, and count a pair as one rep. Do five reps per side.

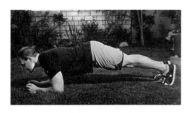

4) Planks (abdominals). Prop yourself on your elbows and toes only, maintaining a rigid torso, ensuring not to let your pelvis dip toward the ground. You will have to contract your abdominals very hard to do this. If you can't hold the position for ten seconds, start on your knees until you can hold that for thirty seconds, and then try the regular version again. Work your way to being able to hold the position for sixty seconds, and add weight to the small of your back with a small plate or dumbbell when that is easy.

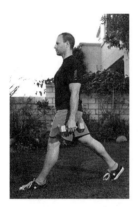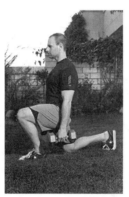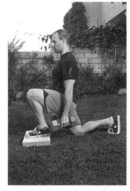

5) Static Lunges (quadriceps, inner thighs, and glutes). Standing with a dumbbell in each hand, get into a lunge position as shown in the first picture. Lunge straight up and straight down from here as shown in the second, keeping a tight arch in your back, and be sure to press through the heel of your front leg. This engages the glutes better. When you have the basic version down, switch to the more advanced version shown to the right where you lunge off a step. You'll get a stronger contraction in your entire thigh and a greater stretch in your hip flexors. Choose a weight that allows you to do ten reps per side.

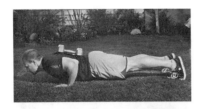

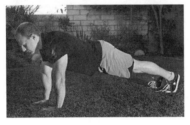

6) Weighted Push-Ups (chest, shoulders, and triceps). Begin with hands next to your body as shown in the picture, looking straight ahead. When doing push-ups, be sure that your stomach doesn't hit the ground before your chest. Stay ramrod straight the entire time! Also, don't let your elbows flare out. Instead keep your arms and elbows close to your body for the entire time. Finally, at the top, really push up as high as possible until your upper back rounds. The second photo shows this without weight to make it easier to see. If you're doing it right, the weight on your back won't fall off as you complete each repetition. If you can't do twelve push-ups, push up from your knees instead of your toes. If you can do more than twelve, place a weight plate on the middle of your back. Choose a weight or method that allows for ten good reps.

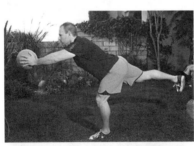

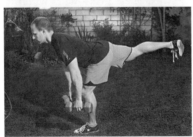

7) Dumbbell Bent-Leg Deadlifts (hamstrings, glutes, and lower back). Begin by holding a medicine ball or other light object in both hands. Now stand on one foot, and as the left picture shows, simultaneously bring the medicine ball out in front of you while kicking one of your legs back. Start by bending your hips, rather than your knees, and tilt forward. Once you've begun the motion with your hips, you can bend your knees slightly. Continue to lower, but stop right before you feel your lower back rounding. Cut the range of motion off before this point. Only go as low on these as you can still maintain the arch in your lower back. You'll know you're doing the movement correctly when you feel your hamstrings stretching as you lower the weight, and your glutes contracting with an arched back. Once you have the hang of this version, switch to dumbbells or kettlebells as shown on the right, choosing a weight for which you can do eight reps. The only difference in movement is that the weights go straight down as the photo shows instead of out front.

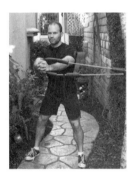

8) Pallof Presses (obliques). This exercise trains the obliques and several other core muscles to resist rotating at the lower back, an essential skill to avoid hurting your spine, not to mention developing killer abs. Start by hooking a band to a post, wall, or tree at chest height. In the photo above, I am holding the cable dead center in my chest, standing perfectly still. The cable is trying to twist my torso straight toward it, but I am resisting that rotational force by holding steady. To make the exercise harder, stick your butt out and bend your knees slightly while always maintaining an arch in your lower back. You can also make it harder by standing farther away from the post or tree. The more you stick your butt out while holding that cable right in line with your breastbone without letting it move you, the more tension you'll feel in your midsection as you resist its pull. Hold for ten seconds at a time, switch sides, and do five more ten-second holds per side.

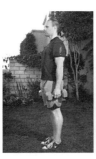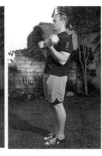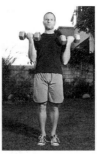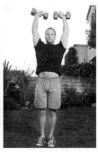

9) Curl and Arnold Dumbbell Overhead Presses (shoulders). This movement has four pictures because it has four parts. While standing, hold two dumbbells at your sides, and curl them forward and up to your shoulders. Make sure your palms are facing you, with the dumbbells held at chest level and close together in their final position. Now push them upward, turning your wrists so that your palms are facing away from you, until your arms are extended over your head. Lower first to your shoulders, and then all the way down. Repeat. Shoot for ten reps.

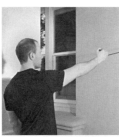

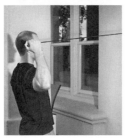

10) Face Pulls (upper back). Place one end of an exercise band in the opening of a door hinge, and close the door so the band stays in place. If your band is a loop, find a small pole or tree you can wrap the loop around, sliding one side of the loop through the other. Adjust the band so that it is perpendicular to the floor when you hold it just above your head. Holding the end of the band, walk away from the door until the band is taut, and your arm is straight out in front of you. Now pull the band toward you and out to the side, so that you finish the motion with your arms in the "hands up" position. Squeeze for one second, and repeat, alternating arms. Perform twelve to fifteen reps.

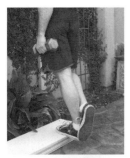

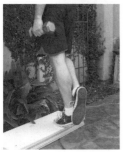

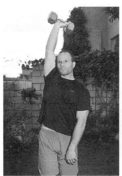

11) Toe Raises (calves). Holding a dumbbell in your right hand, and balancing against a wall with your left, put your right foot at the edge of a step. Allow your heel to drop *slightly* lower than the step as on the left photo above, and then fully extend until you're up on your tippy toes as on the right. Repeat with your left foot once you've completed the set with your right. Do twelve reps.

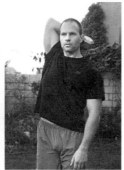

12) One-Arm Overhead Triceps Extensions (triceps). Hold a dumbbell straight over your head, in your right hand. Lower the dumbbell as far as possible behind your head, and then lift it up again. Do all reps for the right side before moving onto the left. Do ten reps.

High-Intensity Interval Training (HIIT) Is a HIT!

What is HIIT? When it comes to "doing cardio to burn fat," this is what really works best. I'll define the concept and give an example first before explaining why. Interval training has many names, but it's generally termed high-intensity cardio or high-intensity interval training (HIIT). Whatever you call it, it's simply defined as performing all-out bursts of activity for twenty to sixty seconds, doing something easy like walking for another twenty to sixty seconds, and then repeating that sequence for a total of ten to fifteen times. That's it. Nothing complicated or fancy. An example would be sprinting for thirty seconds, walking for thirty seconds, and repeating the sequence fourteen more times. While this workout would last only fifteen minutes, it would leave you picking yourself up off the floor, and literally catching your breath for the next twenty-four hours. And that's if you could finish it.

After a quick warm-up by going through the NDP Aerobic Program for one circuit, a typical HIIT workout done with sprints would look like this, preferably done three of the days when you are not lifting weights, or immediately after lifting weights:

- Do one circuit of the New Diabetes Aerobics Program if not lifting weights prior to HIIT.
- Sprint for thirty seconds, and then walk for thirty seconds.
- Repeat fourteen more times for a total of fifteen minutes.
- Stretch for ten to fifteen minutes afterward.

Why is this so effective? The answer lies in why you're "literally catching your breath." Intense forms of exercise like sprinting, a heavy set of squats, fast swimming, or running up stairs are all anaerobic forms of exercise. The translation of "anaerobic" is "without oxygen." Basically, these forms of exercise are so intense that the body cannot use respiration alone (breathing) to sustain the activity. Instead, it has to use stored carbohydrates, creatine, and adenosine triphosphate (ATP) to keep the muscles functioning. ATP and creatine are energy sources used by the body for very short, intense bursts of energy typically lasting less than thirty seconds. A single broad jump or hundred-meter sprint would only use these energy sources. Most anaerobic exercise, including HIIT, will rely on anaerobic glycolysis, a fancy term that describes using both glycogen (stored carbs) and oxygen (breathing) for energy. Even though you use oxygen during HIIT, it's still so intense that you're not getting enough. It is this lack of oxygen that explains why we can't sprint for as long as we can run. However, you have by now noticed that we do need to breathe. And we do need to make up for the oxygen that we couldn't use during the intense exercise. As a result, as soon as the intense bout of exercise is done, the body is in oxygen debt. Exercise physiologists call this state "excess post-exercise oxygen consumption" or EPOC.

EPOC has some wonderful ramifications for weight loss and blood sugar control:

- *It increases growth hormone and other fat-burning hormones*, which coupled with oxygen debt causes more calories to be burned per hour for the next twenty-four to forty-eight hours! Sprinting for fifteen minutes, instead of jogging for an hour, will cause your body to burn an extra 10% to 15% more calories over this time period. There is negligible EPOC after a jog.

- *It increases calories burned from fat*. Normally, calories burned come from several sources: fat, muscle, or glycogen (stored carbohydrates). EPOC causes more total calories to be burned from fat, and most of it burns hours after the bout is over.

- *Any type of exercise that induces EPOC causes hormonal changes that actually increase muscle mass and decrease fat mass*. Runners are lean, but sprinters are muscular as well as lean. The difference is in the way they train. Sprinters do no distance running, and rely primarily on anaerobic exercise for conditioning – jumping, running, weight lifting, and track drills. Marathon runners run long distances, which sacrifices muscle tissue in the process since holding too much muscle on a long run weighs the body down. The lesson is if you want to be lean and muscular, train like the leanest and most muscular – sprinters.

Do you want to lose 30 pounds in one year? Use HIIT, and forget about the excuse of not having enough time. Remember – you don't need to commit large amounts of time to get in shape. Using tools like HIIT, you ensure you're getting the most bang for your buck in terms of exercise that can significantly control blood sugar for long periods of time. You can expect blood pressure and cholesterol to make turns for the better as well.

> In short, high-intensity exercise means your body is doing extra work with less time spent on your part. You must be willing to commit yourself to getting in shape with the time you have.

Perform HIIT with Kettlebell Swings to Spare the Joints!

The high intensity of high-intensity interval training is unsuitable for someone just starting their exercise routine. For example, sprinting, while a fantastic way to do HIIT, just isn't suitable for someone who hasn't exercised in years. You do need some time to get the joints, muscles, and nervous system accustomed to more strenuous activity. Providing you have clearance from your doctor, you can be ready for HIIT in as few as four weeks.

Start by doing the New Diabetes Aerobic Prescription three times a week for three to five circuits, either after your weight lifting, or on the days you're not weight lifting. If you prefer, you may do another form of moderate or low-intensity exercise to prepare yourself for more strenuous activity. After that, you're good to go!

To spare the joints, performing HIIT with kettlebells, bodyweight circuits, or an exercise machine such as an elliptical trainer, stair stepper, or exercise bike are the best options. These forms of exercise require little or no impact on the knees and hips, making them suitable for anyone. In my program, you'll learn to perform an exercise called the swing either with the weight plates you were told to purchase or a kettlebell, which will run you $30 to $50 if you buy it from a sporting goods store (but double that if you have it shipped due to its weight). This simple exercise is best described as swinging the kettlebell or weight plate between your legs as if you are hiking a football, rapidly swinging it forward to chest level, using the power of your hips, and repeating.

A kettlebell is a Russian strength tool that looks like a cannonball with a handle. Over the past few years, they have become extremely popular in the United States thanks to Pavel Tsatsouline, a former Russian kettlebell champion who started the craze here. Kettlebells can be used at home, only take up the space of a basketball, and since they're made of cast iron, will outlast most ice ages. They come in sizes appropriate to anyone. You can order a kettlebell and instructional DVD at http://www.dragondoor.com, or you can make a quick trip to Target.

The swing can be done for intervals, helping you to develop strength and endurance at the same time. The exercise is nonimpact, and can be used even by people with knee, back, or shoulder problems. It develops the glutes to a high degree, and can burn a ton of fat while helping diabetics control blood sugar in a very short amount of time. This makes the swing the best "bang for your buck" HIIT exercise in existence, in my opinion.

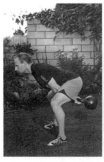 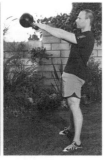

Here I am performing a swing with a kettlebell. I throw the kettlebell between my legs with a clearly arched back, and using the power of my glutes, forcefully thrust it forward. Note the straight line from my arms through the center of the kettlebell on the second picture. This entire rep took less than two seconds. Imagine how much fat gets burned doing 60 to 160 of these!

Learning to Swing a Barbell Plate or Kettlebell

Your first set of swings should be done with a barbell plate and a towel looped through it for a handle. Prior to beginning, go through the entire warm-up, foam rolling, and stretch sequence above. That may be enough of a workout right there for you!

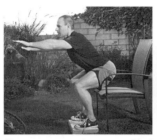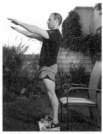

You must absolutely learn to box squat as shown below prior to swinging. The box squat will teach you to sit back with your hips, ensuring you're using your hips and ham-

Box squats must be mastered before trying swings. When done right, you feel your hamstrings and glutes the farther back you sit. Think sit back, not sit down.

strings to swing instead of your quads. It seems simple until you try it. What I'm asking you to do is sit back on a chair as shown, pushing your hips back farther and farther until your butt only slightly touches the chair before standing back up. In other words, don't sit down, rock back in the chair, and then stand up. Instead, just keep shifting your hips back farther and farther until you barely touch the chair. It may help to take a wider stance. If you're doing it right, you'll feel your glutes and hamstrings stretching the farther back you sit. Try doing three sets of five before doing your first set of swings.

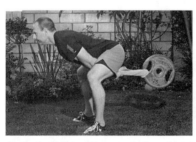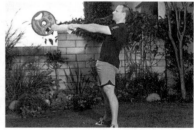

In the first photo, I have pushed my hips back and have a clear arch in my lower back. In the second photo, there is a straight line between my arms, the towel, and the plate, and that line is parallel to the ground.

Once you've got the box squat down, and are pushing back with your hips instead of your quads, you can get into the groove of things with the plate swing. I recommend you do all swings in a vacant area, away from other people who may get hurt if you lose control of the kettlebell or plate while exercising. The plate swing will actually be harder than the normal swing because of the extra degree of freedom where the towel wraps around the plate. There is a very good reason for this: the plate swing will absolutely force you to learn control of the movement faster than words can ever teach you. It will provide instant feedback that will teach you how to get it right. Simply put, you'll know you're doing it wrong if the plate swings wildly high or low instead of keeping in a straight line.

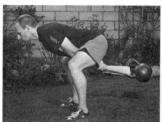
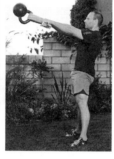

Note the clearly arched lower back and how the hips push back in the first photo. In the second, notice how there is a straight line from arms to towel to kettlebell.

You can continue with plate swings until you get a kettlebell. Once you do, you'll want to continue to practice swinging the kettlebell with a towel as shown above. Once you can consistently swing the kettlebell to above parallel and in a straight line as the second photo above, you may revert to the swing proper from there on out.

That the arms are above parallel means I had used enough power in the hips to get it to that height without compromising form. Once you can do the same, you are good to go with kettlebell swings without a towel from there on out. As a next level of progression, you can try swinging the kettlebell with one arm at a time, eventually switching from hand to hand at the top of the movement.

Ways to Do HIIT

Below are all good ways to perform HIIT. I highly recommend swings, but I want to leave you with several options in case that one is not practical or possible. With all of these, warm up with mobility drills first for five to ten minutes, and then get started. Remember that you're doing this for yourself, and work to surpass your own records, not anyone else's. That's the best way to get a great workout.

- **Kettlebell swings**. The first option here is to swing the kettlebell for thirty seconds, and rest for thirty seconds, repeating the set ten to fifteen times. Another option is to swing the kettlebell for one minute, and rest for four, for a total of four hard minutes. As you advance, move on to more difficult sets. Swing the kettlebell for twenty seconds, and rest for ten, for a total of eight sets, or four minutes of exercise. While it sounds easy, this "Tabata" protocol is one of the most taxing and effective forms of exercise ever encountered. It was originally tested on Japanese Olympic speed skaters, who were left panting when they were done. I do these once or twice a week.

- **Running hills or stairs**. Find hills or stairs that you can run or walk up for thirty to sixty seconds. Get up to the top, walk back down, and repeat the climb ten to fifteen times. Once you can get to the top in less than a minute fifteen times in a row, find a bigger hill or longer set of stairs.

- **High-grade treadmill walk/run.** Set the treadmill to the highest grade possible (or the highest grade you can maintain). Do a hard minute moving as quickly as possible, then lower the speed, but leave the grade level as is. Walk for four minutes, and then repeat the sequence three more times. The total workout looks like this: one hard minute, rest for four minutes, one hard minute, rest for four minutes, one hard minute, rest for four minutes, and one last hard minute. Note: Rest does not mean stop. It means keep moving at a slower pace.

- **Elliptical trainer or exercise bike:** With exercise machines besides the treadmill, I recommend either doing sixty seconds hard followed by four minutes easy for a total of four to five hard minutes, or doing thirty seconds hard and thirty seconds easy for a total of fifteen hard intervals.

Chart Your Workouts in Your Journal

The more muscle you build, and the more fat you burn, the more diabetes improves. But how do you know when you've made progress with an exercise? Is it when you can do more weight? What if you can do more reps with the same weight or less rest? These are all signs that you're improving, but are you going to remember all of that? Are you going to be able to remember all of those numbers over the next six months? Probably not. The only people who ever make progress in the gym are those who know what progress they've made. That's why you're going to download an exercise journal from my website, http://www.TheNewDiabetesPrescription.com. Follow this outline every time you work out. Fill it out at the end or while exercising. Do this *every time* you work out. It doesn't have to be complicated, and it doesn't have to take a lot of time. It does need to be done. The sheet below will help you keep track of

- Order of exercises.
- Number of sets, reps, and rest between sets.
- Total weight of all sets on all exercises.
- Total workout time and date of workout.
- Amount, type, length, and perceived difficulty of any cardiovascular exercise.
- How you felt at the end, and any notes you have about the exercises (how to perform better, ease, discomfort, etc.).

When you become more advanced, you can make a workout journal of your own. But this example will do for now. My own workout journal takes me about five minutes to update. Those five minutes make a profound difference on the next forty to sixty minutes I spend exercising. It's a very simple but powerful tool. A workout journal not only lets you see whether you're making progress in an exercise but also whether you can do more reps or the same workout in less time (which is a way to increase fitness). It's not al-

THE NEW DIABETES PRESCRIPTION FOR EXERCISE DAILY JOURNAL

Foam roll upper & lower legs, back, and chest, and stretch
before beginning – it takes 5 minutes.

#	Go through once before weights, 3 times for low-intensity cardio
1	3x5 Reps of Ankle Mobilizations per Leg
2	5 Reps of Knee-Ups per Leg
3	5 Reps of Cradle Walks per Leg
4	5 Reps of Butt Kicks per Leg
5	10 Reps of Leg Swings per Leg
6	3x5 Reps of 3-D Lunges per Leg
7	10 Reps of Spider Mans
8	10 Reps of Glute Bridges per Leg

#	Exercise Pairs (Do each exercise with the same letter back to back without rest)	Weight
A1	Mini-Band Side Steps	
A2	Super Bird Dogs	
B1	Side Bridges	
B2	Planks	
C1	Static Lunges	
C2	Push-Ups	
D1	Dumbbell Deadlifts	
D2	Pallof Presses	
E1	Dumbbell Curl & Overhead Press	
E2	Face Pulls	
F1	Toe Raises	
F2	Overhead Triceps Extensions	

HIIT: KETTLEBELL OR PLATE SWINGS WITH A TOWEL

Add 1 set of 10 swings every other workout. Once you can do 10 sets of 10 reps,
drop to 5 sets of 12 and build up to 10 sets of 12. Drop to 5 sets of 14
until you reach 10 sets of 14 and so on.

#	THE NEW DIABETES PRESCRIPTION FOR EXERCISE DAILY JOURNAL	
#	Go through once before weights, 3 times for low-intensity cardio	
9	10 Reps of C-Clams per Leg	
10	8 Reps of Two-Legged Deadlifts per Leg	
11	5 Reps of One-Legged Deadlifts per Leg	
12	3x5 Reps of Thoracic Extensions	
13	3x5 Reps of Thoracic Rotations	
14	10 Reps of Push-Ups	
15	12 Reps of Scapular Rotations per Arm	
16	10 Reps of Wall Slides	

Reps for Set 1	Rest for Set 1	Reps for Set 2	Rest for Set 2	Reps for Set 3	Rest for Set 3

	Fill in how many reps per set you did below				
	SET 1	SET 2	SET 3	SET 4	SET 5

ways an advanced technique or esoteric piece of knowledge that gets you ahead - often it is doing the simple things that you should have been doing all along.

Seeing the Progress

For those of you who think you hate exercise, think again. Like a battery between charges, your body – and your mindset – may seem to eschew working out. But an active lifestyle can replace an entire pharmacy. It can get you out of pain. It can give you back your life. And within a few days, it begins to feel really good.

Progress with exercise is a broad term for a diabetic. Monitor not only the scale, but how your blood sugar is going down, and if you need to cut back on medication. Those are two major benefits and victories for you. How are your blood pressure, cholesterol, and energy improving?

The scale may very well be the last number to go down, but I don't want you to take that as a bad thing. Since you'll be gaining muscle and losing fat simultaneously, the tightness of your clothes may change before the scale does. Since one pound of muscle takes up one-fifth of the space of one pound of fat, the best way to see progress is to measure your body parts in inches every week, and track those changes along with the scale. The scale-and-tape-measure combination will give you a true testimony as to how your body is changing. And be prepared for variations: you'll see more change some weeks and less others. But those who succeed in the end are the ones who keep doing right by themselves during the weeks when nothing happens. Persistence is required to win at this game.

Pay particular attention to your waist measurement, where the toxin-spouting visceral fat is stored. Of all the places you could lose weight that will have the greatest impact on your health, this is where you want to lose it. Below forty inches for men and thirty-five inches for women is a great start. This fat is very metabolically active, so you may find losing it to actually be fairly quick once you get going on your diet and exercise routine. When it's gone, the majority of the fat around your middle will be the run-of-the-mill subcutaneous fat. That will take more work, but every inch lost will mean lower blood sugar, cholesterol, and blood pressure for the rest of your life.

The Fourth Prescription in Summary

- Exercise causes weight loss, reduces blood pressure, blood cholesterol, and blood sugar. It fights every aspect of metabolic syndrome, and can work as well as medication.

- Exercise lessens the amount of insulin needed to transport glucose into your cells. It can process glucose independent of insulin.

- You must make room for exercise in your life. And twenty minutes of walking cut into 4 five-minute sessions a day *ain't* going to cut it! You need about 300 minutes a week to truly change your life.

- Move an hour a day. Even if you can't go through the exercises given above for a whole sixty minutes, walk, bike, or use another exercise machine until sixty minutes are up. You will make progress.

- Use a foam roller on your tight muscles to alleviate pain and make exercise easier and more effective.

- You will get a fantastic cardiovascular workout by going through the mobility drills listed above in three to five circuits. Besides burning calories, you feel better, you will move better, and you will have less pain.

- Do your cardio after weight training or on days when you don't weight train. When ready, add HIIT to your cardio routine or replace it with HIIT. Kettlebell swings are ideal here.

- You must weight train three days per week on nonconsecutive days.

FIFTH PRESCRIPTION

Follow A Low-Carb Diet *Most Of The Time...*

*Y*ou will want to follow a low-carb diet with periodic breaks that will let you eat old favorites but still lose fat. Why? A low-carb diet can be defined many ways, but here, it is defined as eating fewer than thirty grams of carbohydrates per day. A low-carb diet does *not* mean never having your favorite desserts again. It does *not* mean eating only meat and cheese. It certainly does not mean you go low carb and don't exercise. Exercise will do as much for stopping insulin resistance as following a low-carb diet. It does mean eating plenty of fish, chicken, eggs, beef, nuts, seeds, vegetables, dairy, legumes, some fruits, and some starches.

I want to be very clear with you. There are some of us who will never be able to eat and metabolize as many carbs as others. As a type II diabetic, if you're really interested in losing weight, reducing or eliminating meds, and regaining your health, you will never be able to eat as many carbs as your starch-obsessed rail-thin relative, friend, or coworker. The reason, you'll recall, is insulin resistance.

- Insulin resistance is the reason you're a diabetic.
- Insulin resistance is the reason why your friends can lose weight on complex-carb diets and you can't.
- Insulin resistance is the reason why your scale stops moving way short of your weight-loss goal.
- Insulin resistance is the reason why you carry the bulk of your fat around your middle, regardless of your gender.

Two individuals, one insulin resistant and one not, even with the same activity level, gender, muscle mass, and weight, will process the same meal completely differently. The noninsulin resistant person will store far less of her meals as fat. She can eat more calories and not gain weight. She can lose weight faster. Meanwhile, the insulin-resistant individual will have problems losing weight even from too many good sources of carbohydrates like apples and brown rice. Forget fast food! How bad is it if you can't even lose weight eating a freaking apple!

> **As a type II diabetic, even an appropriately sized healthy lunch of chicken breast, brown rice, and steamed spinach can be a problem.**

Healthy starches and fruits will still raise your blood sugar more than low-carb foods, and they also get in the way of what a low-carb diet without them can do for you.

Protein requires much less insulin to process while fat requires nearly zero. By eating a lower-carb diet, your body will need less insulin, making fat burning possible again. I'm not saying never pop another French fry in your mouth. But carbohydrates raise your blood sugar the most, are the most often abused, and for a diabetic, lay on the most fat.

Low-carb dieting's profound effect on fat loss has already been made popular by the late Dr. Robert Atkins in his book, *The Dr. Atkins New Diet Revolution.* Study after study has vindicated his claim that eating more fat and fewer carbs burns fat and treats every single aspect of the metabolic syndrome[3].

Low-carb diets even protect the heart against bad cholesterol better than low-fat diets[2]. In fact, studies have shown cholesterol on a low-carb diet improves even when large amounts of saturated fat are consumed, even when there is no weight loss. Low-fat diets on the other hand seem to need weight loss to get a similar effect (cholesterol usually goes down as people lose weight).[6] I personally consume over 100 grams of fat per day, most of it monounsaturated omega-3s, the magical fat found in fish and some nuts. My cholesterol is perfect: a very low 42 mg/dl triglycerides (bad cholesterol) and a very high 89 mg/dl HDL (good cholesterol). Restricting carbohydrates improves all aspects of the metabolic syndrome[3] of which high blood sugar is only one small part.

The First Way Low-Carb Diets Kill the Killer —Less Hunger and More Calories Burned

After a protein and fat meal like a steak, you're likely to feel fuller after three hours than after having a calorically equivalent amount of rice. Within two weeks of following a low-carb diet in one study, obese diabetics voluntarily reduced their food intake because they felt less hungry. Even better, their glucose, insulin levels, triglycerides, cholesterol, hA1c, and insulin resistance all improved[4].

Several studies now point out that higher-protein diets "lead to a higher decrease of energy intake at the next meal than carbohydrate and fat. A protein-enriched diet induces satiety, improves body composition and results in weight loss."[36] One reason given for the satiety effect of protein is that it increases cholecystokinin (CCK), a stomach hormone that reduces hunger. Another reason is that ghrelin levels remain depressed longer following meals higher in protein and fat than carbohydrates[34-35]. You may recall from the First Prescription that when the hormone ghrelin elevates, hunger increases, and leptin levels in the brain drop[33].

Interestingly, one reason overweight people have a hard time getting full on high-carb foods is that their stomachs depress ghrelin *less* after a high-carb meal compared to leaner individuals[37]. This surprised researchers who were expecting the opposite to happen. Instead, they found their overweight test subjects consumed nearly half the number of calories eating meat compared to those who ate bread. In other words, if you have a lot of weight to lose, you're going to feel like eating fewer calories going low-carb than high carb.

You can also get away with eating more calories and still lose fat! Several studies have shown low-carb diets lose an extra 5.5 pounds over twelve weeks compared to low-fat dieters[5]. That equates on average to an extra 230 calories burned per day.

In another study where normal-weight men went on a low-carb diet with enough calories to maintain body weight, they still wound up losing an average 7.5 pounds of fat, and gaining nearly 2.5 pounds of muscle[14]. The researchers determined the bulk of the fat loss was attributable to the 34% measured drop in insulin levels, and somewhat due to slightly increased T4 thyroid hormone levels. A five pound change in body-weight over six weeks equates to an extra 243 calories burned per day, significantly close to what the other study measured.

When forty-five obese subjects were fed either a 1,000 calorie-per-day high-fat or high-carb diet for thirty days, the low carbers lost an average of 9.2 more pounds[15]. That equates to burning an extra 1,073 calories per day *more* than the high-carb group! Your own mileage may vary of course, but a low-carb diet's effects on fat loss will still be greater than if you followed a higher-carb, lower-fat diet.

Now, for someone who may have found it impossible to ever lose a pound, you can appreciate finally being able to feel full after a meal while still losing weight.

Feeling neither hunger nor lack of energy is a huge psychological boost.

This really is a strategy that will allow you to lose the weight.

The Second Way Low-Carb Diets Kill the Killer —Better Blood Pressure and Cholesterol

Since your liver is no longer trying to turn every carbohydrate and fat molecule that comes its way into body fat and cholesterol, your LDL cholesterol (the bad one) will go down, and your HDL cholesterol (the good one) will rise.

> In one study, twenty-nine men following a low-carb diet lost 16.5 pounds, dropped their LDL 8.9% and their triglycerides 38.6%, and increased their HDL by 12%[7].

Low-carb diets are not only great for lowering body fat and blood sugar, but great for your blood pressure and cholesterol.[1] Its diuretic, insulin-lowering, and heart-helpful effects will drop your blood pressure[8-11]. With a few supplements, exercise, and weight loss, you may eventually be able to get off your blood pressure meds altogether!

The Third Way Low-Carb Diets Kill the Killer —Enhanced Fat Burning and Muscle Building

By eating meals high in fat, moderate in protein, and low in carbs, metabolic pathways responsible for burning fat go into high gear, allowing your body to use fat from your diet and body for fuel instead of glucose. You might recall that HSL, the enzyme that breaks down body fat, is better able to do its job of releasing fat from stores when insulin levels are under control. On a low-carb diet, these freed fatty acids are better used for energy in the absence of carbohydrate.

> As your body starts to use your own fat stores for energy, you lose weight. You eat fat without carbs so your body will start burning its own fat!

The burning of body fat on a low-carb diet is termed lipolysis, and is different than ketosis, which occurs when eating under thirty grams of carbs per day. While ketosis is unnecessary for fat loss and blood sugar control, you'll be eating fewer than thirty grams of carbs per day on the low-carb portion of the diet to ensure maximum lipolysis.

Low-carb dieting also works because it preserves muscle mass better than low-fat dieting. In one study, the more fat and fewer carbs rats were fed, the more fat they lost and muscle they gained[12]. When obese women were put on a high-protein, low-carb diet or a high-carb, low-protein diet with equal calories for ten weeks, the low carbers lost significantly more fat and less muscle than the high carbers.[13]

After a diet, you are only as lean as the fat you lost and the muscle you kept.

The Fourth Way Low-Carb Diets Kill the Killer —Improved Insulin Sensitivity

Check out the results from this study in which forty patients with atherogenic dyslipidemia (hardened arteries and bad cholesterol) went on a low-carb diet for twelve weeks:

- They lowered their blood sugar by 12%.
- They cut blood insulin levels in half and improved insulin sensitivity by 55%.
- They lost 10% of their body weight, including 14% body fat.
- They lowered triglycerides 51% and improved their good HDL by 13%[1].

As I stated earlier, with less insulin required to process your foods, your pancreas gets a rest. Over time, a poor functioning pancreas may begin to function so much better that you may no longer need insulin or oral hypoglycemics when you do ingest carbohydrates (remember you'll be following a low-carb diet most of the time—not all of the time). With less insulin knocking on the door of your cells, they too get a much-needed break to rejuvenate and repair their insulin receptors. As the low-carb diet drops body fat, and your pancreas and cells repair, you become less and less insulin resistant, less and less type II diabetic.

A Low-Carb Diet Is a High-Fat Diet. . . and *That's Not Bad*

> **Fat is critical to your success on a low-carb diet.**
> **You need fat to burn fat. Fat is your friend.**

Even saturated fat can be beneficial. Multiple studies have confirmed replacing carbohydrates in the diet for dietary fat improves cardiovascular risk factors instead of hindering them[16]. In fact, researchers found twenty-eight obese men who included eggs in their diet for twelve weeks had higher HDL levels and better markers for heart health than obese low carbers taking an egg substitute[17-18]. The researchers attributed the results to the cholesterol in eggs. Low fat with high protein does not give these benefits.

Why Low-Carb Meal Plans Really Work. . .

By eating fat-burning proteins and cholesterol-killing fats, you're *not* eating crackers, cereal, cakes, bagels, cookies, candy, pasta, French fries, beer, or pizza – the foods that honestly cause obesity, diabetes, high cholesterol, high blood pressure, and heart disease.

If you're cutting carbs, you're not downing oversized portions of crappy foods laden with sugar and refined flour.

> **80% of fat loss comes from what you**
> *don't* **put in your mouth!**

Think about that above statement – low carbers immediately adopt the habit of cutting out all refined carbohydrate-and-sugar-laden foods and beverages. This is a habit that everyone who is lean adheres to more than 90% of the time. Ninety percent of their meals do not include these foods, and the 10% that do are not huge portion sizes!

The New Diabetes Low-Carb Prescription

1. Cut your carbs to thirty grams or less for every low-carb day. Don't shoot for zero carbs, but it's vital you stay under thirty. You will go off the low-carb diet for one to two days every five to twelve days as explained below.

2. This is a high-fat, medium-protein, low-carb diet. This is not a high-protein, low-fat, low-carb diet. Get 55 to 60% of your calories from fat. None of it can come from trans-fatty acids (check the food label).

3. Drink nothing but tea, coffee, sparkling water, and water. No alcohol! If you must have them, keep diet sodas down to two or fewer per day. Avoid too many carbonated beverages because the carbonation leaches calcium from your system.

4. Do not count fiber as a carbohydrate. Subtract it from the carb totals in foods.

5. No matter what a food package says, count all sugar alcohols (glycerol, erythritol, sorbitol, mannitol, xylitol, and maltitol) as a gram of carbohydrate. Sugar alcohols will be clearly marked as carbohydrates under the total carbohydrate count under the food's nutritional information.

6. Avoid having artificial sweetener – too much will stop fat burning. If you must have it, have no more than four packets in a day. Count each packet of artificial sweetener as one carb. Choose Stevia over Splenda, Splenda over Sweet'n Low, Sweet'n Low over Equal, and Equal over sugar.

Low-Carb Eating Is Hard for the First Two Weeks, but Then It Gets Easy!

You may experience a plethora of carb withdrawal symptoms during the first two weeks of the diet which will eventually subside including headaches, sugar and starch cravings, insomnia, irritability, feeling spaced out, constipation, and fatigue. Constipation is relieved with green leafy vegetables, nuts, flaxseeds, glucomannan, and psyllium husks. Headaches, insomnia, irritability, and carb cravings will disappear with 5-HTP. Glutamine will also help with cravings. Fatigue will disappear in a few days.

> ## The first two weeks are tough. The next two decades are a lot easier.

Because carbs are involved in proper bowel movements, you can expect some constipation. This is why you *must* use low-carb fiber supplements such as psyllium husks (found in Metamucil), glucomannan powder, and ground flaxseeds. You can also have as many of these high-fiber, low-carb vegetables as you want: watercress, broccoli, turnips, spinach, asparagus, cucumbers, and romaine lettuce. While you should be eating a lot of fibrous green vegetables like spinach, broccoli, brussels sprouts, asparagus, and romaine lettuce, you'll still come up short in the fiber department. Fiber is essential for detoxification and fat loss. It helps regulate insulin levels and adds to fullness. You'll lose weight faster and be healthier in the long term if you include it.

Again, all of these symptoms will subside after the two-week mark. Once your body has adjusted, you'll feel better than you've felt in years. Your cravings will be gone. Your blood sugar will be the most stable of your entire diabetic life. Your energy will high. You'll get up in the morning easier. But, again, the first two weeks will be hard.

If you are a type I diabetic, ketones in your urine are a problem only if your blood sugar is sky high. If you find ketones in your urine, and your blood sugar is 90 mg/dl, don't call an ambulance. However, do make sure your glucometer is working! If so, it's benign dietary ketosis, and *not* diabetic ketoacidosis.

Your doctor will need to know that you are starting a low-carb diet so she can regulate your blood sugar prescription medications. The combination may be too much, resulting in low blood sugar. Keep checking your fasting and postprandial blood sugars to see your progress and to check for hypoglycemia. If you start getting hypoglycemia, take your glucose tabs, evaluate when and what you last ate, and talk to your doctor about lowering your diabetic meds. *Do not* let yourself walk around in a hypoglycemic cloud because you *falsely* believe you'll ruin your diet by popping some glucose tabs. Indeed, you're actually helping it *in this state*. So there is no reason for guilt, and no reason to not *immediately* treat your low blood sugar.

If you are exercising intensely, and you at any time on this diet experience the symptoms of hypoglycemia (sweating, shaking, disorientation, dizziness, sugar cravings, irritability, brain fog, heart pounding), then you need to sip some carbs while exercising. Mix glucose tablets (or pure dextrose) with a scoop of protein powder, and sip this over an hour-long exercise session. Increase the amounts *slightly* as needed.

Taking a Break from Your Low-Carb Diet Helps the Killer Of Killers Kill Better

If low-carb dieting is so great for diabetes and weight loss, you're probably wondering why I would ever want you to take a break from it. The short answer is because we can do better. You can lose fat faster, control cravings better, have more energy, and build more muscle taking one- to two-day breaks from your low-carb diet every five to ten days because carbohydrates raise leptin. A break is defined as eating far more than thirty grams of carbohydrates from high-quality sources, the exact number you'll learn later. For now, accept that you'll be periodically taking a break from low-carb eating. This break can also coincide with special occasions and holidays so you don't feel like you're depriving yourself of your favorite treats.

High-fat diets and low-calorie diets both lower leptin in the long run, but increasing calories and carb loading bring leptin levels back up[21]. In men and women given equal calorie meals either high in fat or carbohydrate, the high-carb group had the highest leptin levels afterward[20]. The advantages of keeping leptin up for a dieter are numerous:

- Fewer weight loss stalls.
- Far fewer cravings.
- More energy.
- Muscle growth.
- Faster metabolism.
- Far less chance of rebounding from weight loss.

After eating fewer than thirty carbs for at least three days, your muscles' glycogen stores, where carbohydrates are stored for fuel, are only filled to 50% of their maximum capacity. This makes intuitive sense – if the body is not being fed carbs for fuel, its stores of carbs will be lower. However, if you were to all of a sudden take in a lot of complex carbohydrates in this depleted state, you could fill those glycogen stores back up without putting on any fat, even though you're insulin resistant! You could do this for up to two full days before your muscle glycogen stores became full again. Carbs are used for fuel or stored as muscle glycogen first, and stored as fat second. If there is a place for those carbs to go before they reach your fat cells, they will go there.

Bodybuilders, fitness enthusiasts, and athletes have been using these low-carb/high-carb diets for years, generally termed a Cyclic Carbohydrate Diet (CCD), because you are indeed cycling your carbohydrates week to week. On a CCD, the individual cuts their carbs to less than thirty grams for five days, while getting anywhere from 25 to 35% of their calories from protein, and the rest fat. Experts will argue for the pros and cons of getting more or less protein, but this is the general range. Then, the individual carb loads for a period of 24 to 48 hours. Ideally, the total calories taken in during this time are only 25% higher than one's maintenance level. During this time, the muscles supersaturate with glycogen, and new muscle is built. Then, the individual goes right back to a low-carb diet for five days, once again depleting their carbs, and once again losing fat. Ideally, this type of diet will build the greatest amount of muscle and burn the greatest amount of fat. Exercising only makes this more effective.

Ingesting carbohydrates after following a low-carb diet for five to six days increases fat burning while eating carbs[39-40]. This is partially because hormone-sensitive lipase, the enzyme responsible for breaking down body fat, is elevated as much as 20%[41].

And let's be honest—being able to eat carbs without laying on fat is only the first advantage of clean carb loading. You also get a psychological break when you can occasionally indulge in usually forbidden foods, albeit in moderation. The result is more energy, less fat, and a way to not gain weight from Christmas dinner. Your low-carb diet winds up working as well on week 100 as it did on week 1, and you don't have to give up eating carbs. In contrast, when you eat carbs all the time, you get nothing but fat gain and poor blood sugar control!

> **Cycling your carbohydrates is the best deal you're going to get. You are forbidden nothing, and nearly any food can help you lose fat when eaten at the right time. You simply must be willing to partition your high-carb foods for the weekends instead of the weekdays to benefit, and you must select mostly quality carb sources.**

That's it. Fruits, vegetables, legumes and whole grains are the mainstay here. Complex carbs like oats, potatoes, and wild rice are the most important since they fill up glycogen stores the most. In the Sixth Prescription, you'll learn more about which carbohydrates to choose, and which ones to run from.

How Often to Carb Load, And How Many Carbs to Eat

Research has shown an elite endurance athlete could carb load with up to 4.5 grams for every lean pound of body weight per day, but the glycemic index (how much it raises blood sugar) of the carbs does matter[38]. I don't know about you, but I am not an elite endurance athlete. At my weight and percentage of body fat, this strategy would have me ingesting over 600 grams of carbs per day! Hello diabetic coma...

An appropriate-sized carb load for a diabetic starts by establishing your BMI: Weight (lb) $\times$ 703 $\div$ Height^2 (in^2). Although this formula can be grossly inaccurate in weight lifters, the BMI is an excellent tool in a diabetic population for determining how much weight you need to lose.

> **The more weight you need to lose, the less tolerant your body is going to be to carbohydrates. Carb loading is a game of not too much and not too little. If you don't take in enough carbs from time to time, your metabolism can stall, which we do not want. However, if you overdo it, you'll wind up gaining weight.**

Therefore, the higher your BMI is, the more insulin resistant you probably are, and the less total carbs we want you to have right now.

If Your BMI Is 30 or More

1. You will carb load for one to two days after ten to twelve days of low-carb dieting (e.g., every other weekend).

2. If for over two days, have 0.3 grams of carbohydrate per pound of body weight each day.

3. If you've scheduled your carb load for a holiday or other special occasion, you may have 0.6 grams of carbohydrate per pound of body weight on this one day. Go back to your low-carb diet the next day.

4. If you would like to eat the maximum number of carbs without gaining or losing any weight, shoot for 20% of your total calories from carbohydrate. The Eighth Prescription will help you determine how many calories and carbohydrates that is.

5. You may have one cheat meal per carb load. The rest of your carbs *must* come from fruits, vegetables, legumes, and some whole grains.

6. Include fiber and protein with each high-carb meal to blunt blood sugar.

If Your BMI Is Less Than 30

1. You will carb load for one to two days after five days of low-carb dieting (e.g., every weekend).

2. If done over two days, have 0.6 grams of carbohydrate per pound of body weight on day one, and 0.3 grams per pound of body weight on day two.

3. If you've scheduled your carb load for a holiday or other special occasion, you may have 0.9 grams of carbohydrate per pound of body weight on this one day. Go back to your low-carb diet the next day.

4. If you would like to eat the maximum number of carbs without gaining or losing any weight, shoot for 40% of your total calories from carbohydrate. The Eighth Prescription will help you determine how many calories and carbohydrates that is.

5. You may have one cheat meal per carb load. The rest of your carbs *must* come from fruits, vegetables, legumes, and some whole grains.

6. Include fiber and protein with each high-carb meal to blunt blood sugar.

How to Not Screw Up the Carb Load

Due to the preciseness of what's asked of you, you'll have to plan this carb load in advance. That is quite intentional. You will lose weight and control your emotional eating because you will know beforehand what you're going to eat, and what impact that food will have on your body. If you're going to have a cheeseburger and fries, you'll have to know how many carbs are in that meal beforehand. To track your favorite foods, go to the website of where they're sold, or visit http://www.nutritiondata.com.

Monitor your blood sugar very carefully during the clean carb phase. It is a guarantee that your blood sugar will fluctuate more during the carb-loading period than the low-carb period. It is vital that it does not go too high. Check your blood sugar around ninety minutes after eating, and shoot for a postprandial blood sugar of less than 160 mg/dl. In the Eighth Prescription, you'll learn how supplements like Gymnema sylvestre, vanadyl sulfate, and alpha lipoic acid can help eat up extra sugar. This may be the only time you need to use them.

Getting the prescribed number of carbohydrates is not written in stone. You may tolerate far more carbohydrates with great success, or you may need fewer carbs than this. However, these estimates, and they are estimates, are a great place to start. Pay attention to the signs of too many carbs: carb cravings, water retention, bloating, puffiness, fatigue, and, ultimately, fat gain. This point will occur somewhere on the second day, or after your first cheat meal if you've overdone it. When that time arrives, go back to the low-carb menu! At this point, you're no longer benefiting from the carb load.

The New Diabetes Prescription Diet's Secret Weapon: Fish Oil

Besides carb loading, fish oil is the second major way you will manipulate leptin. One amazing study showed insulin-resistant rats living on a high sugar diet, but supplementing with fish oil, had 70% higher leptin levels compared to a control group, and didn't gain weight despite eating more calories per day[22]! Compare that to the previous study that showed only a 40% increase in leptin from massive overfeeding. This makes fish oil a vital way to keep your metabolic rate elevated as leptin levels drop from decreases in body fat and carbohydrate.

In another compelling study, scientists tried to make fifty-four mice as fat as possible over thirteen weeks. Apart from the mice that did not gain a lot of weight, the rest had very high markers for leptin resistance. Several were then placed on a high-fat diet rich in fish oil, or a low-fat diet. While both the low-fat and high-in-fish-oil diets helped the mice lose all of their weight, only those fed fish oil actually reversed their markers for leptin resistance. When the scientists fed fish oil to already obese mice, they too reversed their markers for leptin resistance[23]. Fish oil is the real deal.

Mice fed a diet of 20% fish oil had 50 to 60% less fat than those fed a diet with the same number of calories without fish oil[42]. The researchers concluded the fish oil slowed the growth of fat cells, and increased fat burning[42-43]. Don't you think you want this in your diet!?

And the results don't stop at mice. When prediabetic human subjects consumed a diet with 20% monounsaturated fats, they had a better fasting glucose and did better on a glucose challenge test than prediabetics fed polyunsaturated fats[19].

But really, the benefits of fish oil extend so far beyond just controlling leptin and losing fat. Fish oil helps every aspect of diabetes. In fact, if I could choose only one supplement to use for the rest of my life, it'd be the fish oil.

Over 20,000 doctors who ate fatty fish like salmon at least once per week over eleven years were found to be half as likely to have a fatal cardiac event than those who ate fish once per month or not at all[51]. Fish oils lower triglycerides, LDL cholesterol, and arterial platelet collection[44], avoiding the formation of blood clots. It's also essential to making heart cells more elastic, helping the heart return to resting state more easily, thereby avoiding arrhythmias[44]. These results led the researchers to conclude that "fish oil has demonstrated reductions in risk that compare favorably with those seen in landmark secondary prevention trials with lipid-lowering drugs."[44]

In another study, fifty-nine patients with heart disease who took two grams per day of a pharmaceutical-grade fish oil lowered triglycerides 20% to 30% and very low-density lipoprotein 30% to 40%.[45]

Whether your kidneys have already been damaged from diabetes, or you're at risk (and as a diabetic, you are), fish oil can help. Fish oil reduced the urine calcium levels of patients on dialysis with kidney stones[51]. Other patients on dialysis required one-sixth less erythropoietin and had nearly a 4% lower level of albumin compared to a placebo[52]. In those at risk of kidney disease, fish oil slowed nephropathy[51]. And 4,000 mg of fish oil was shown to be very powerful at lowering blood pressure[46-50].

While getting your omega-3s will greatly assist you in all the above areas, not getting them will be to your *significant detriment in those areas*. Nearly everyone on earth is not getting enough of the fat found in fish, namely omega-3 fatty acids. It's an essential fatty acid (EFA) because you must get them from food. Your body cannot make them, and they are involved in just about every bio-chemical process you can imagine. By including them daily, you'll have fewer stalls, more energy, and less hunger when trying to lose weight by including omega-3s in your diet, even if that slightly increases your total daily calories. It's these little decisions that sometimes net big payoffs in the diabetes and fat-loss game.

Omega-3s come in three forms (get ready): alpha-linolenic acid (ALA), eicosapentaenoic acid (EPA), and docosahexaenoic acid (DHA). They are found in:

- Salmon, tuna, mackerel, sardine, herring, anchovies, caviar, and other cold water fish.
- Fish oil capsules and regular fish oil made from any of the above fish.
- Walnuts and butter nuts.
- Flaxseed oil and milled flaxseeds.
- Seaweed, peppers, radishes, beans, spinach, cauliflow-er, brussels sprouts, squash, kale, and broccoli.
- Tofu.

You may also read linolenic acid on a food label, meaning Omega-3.

EPA and DHA are the two omega-3 fatty acids found in fish oil. The third omega-3, alpha-linolenic acid (ALA), abundant in flaxseeds, has a host of benefits all its own. ALA lowers blood pressure and LDL cholesterol[53]. It also boosts immunity and fights inflammation.

Flaxseeds are great for diabetics beyond their rich content in ALA. Two tablespoons of milled flaxseeds have nearly three grams of ALA, four grams of fiber, and three grams of complete protein, meaning it can be used by the body without needing to add other foods. It also helps regulate estrogen levels, fights cancer, and goes great in smoothies, yogurt, cottage cheese, and salads. We use flaxseeds in the *New Diabetes Prescription* for its impact on blood pressure and cholesterol and for its high fiber content.

What flax can't do is be a substitute for fish oil. It only contains ALA, not the omega-3s EPA and DHA found in fish. Instead, some of the ALA is later converted to DHA and EPA at a very low rate – as little as one gram of DHA and EPA for every six grams of ALA. Also, flax oil has none of the fiber or protein, and can go rancid in the bottle. Stick to the seeds for your health benefits.

Fish is the best source of EPA and DHA. Three and a half ounces of salmon has about 1.5 grams of these marine lipids. Salmon oil capsules will have 200 mg to around 600 mg of EPA and DHA per tablet, and while more portable than fish oil, they are not as cost effective compared to the oil form. For example, one tablespoon of highly concentrated fish oil has up to four grams of EPA and DHA in the twelve grams of fat per tablespoon. I happily pay every three weeks for my bottle of Carlson Lab's Very Finest Fish Oil. If you can't afford fish oil, start eating salmon, tuna, mackerel, sardines, herring, anchovies, caviar, and other cold water fish.

I recommend you get a minimum of 4,000 mg from a combination of EPA plus DHA and four tablespoons of milled flaxseeds daily. Fish oil can be found relatively cheap online at places like http://www.vitacost.com, and a month's supply of flaxseeds should cost less than $5, available in most health food and grocery stores.

Six EPA and DHA grams is the more effective dosage for aggressively treating all the facets of the metabolic syndrome. Don't just go after one symptom of diabetes – go after the cause!

You should not get all of this in one meal, instead spreading out the dose to two or three different meals. Feel free to also get oleic acid, the heart-healthy fat found in olive oil, along with this Prescription. Olive oil is rich in phenols, a type of antioxidant that can increase the elasticity of arterial walls, decreasing the chance of stroke and heart attack. Consuming olive oil also decreases blood pressure and cholesterol, making it fine to cook with and to use in salad dressings. By all means, have at it along with your omega-3s!

Flax has a nice nutty taste and goes well on salads and in shakes. Most fish oils are flavored with lemon, completely eliminating the fishy taste, also making them perfect for dressings, shakes, or even to just be downed by the tablespoon. Because omega-3s can go rancid quickly, be sure your bottles of fish and flax oil are opaque, refrigerate them immediately upon opening, and use them within sixty days from that point.

Other Ways The New Diabetes Prescription Manipulates Leptin

The amino acid 5-HTP may also be beneficial during the low-carb phase of the diet. While 5-HTP's ability to kill sugar cravings has already been touted, studies show it may also raise leptin levels by increasing insulin[24-25]. 5-HTP might be just the ticket if you find your carb cravings increasing the day or days just before you begin another carb load. I sometimes get this, and 5-HTP plus fish oil in my protein shakes takes the sensations completely away. I suggest adding 50 to 100 mg of 5-HTP two to three times per day if needed.

Simply avoiding high-fructose corn syrup and high-glycemic refined carbohydrates may be the simplest way to improve leptin levels. While this won't be a problem following the low-carb portion of the diet, you must be aware of how much damage these foods have already done to you.

High-glycemic carbohydrates significantly decrease leptin levels and increase blood sugar and glucose levels[26]. That's a pretty bad one-two punch for fat loss. In the short term, high blood sugar and insulin will lay on fat. In the long run, leptin lowers, decreasing your metabolism with it.

Fructose, unlike glucose, does not raise blood sugar levels, so it doesn't raise insulin levels, and it doesn't raise leptin levels. So it's not really correct to say all carbohydrates raise leptin. It's more correct to say "all carbs except fructose."[27] Leptin is your brain's way of determining how many calories you've eaten each day. It's what keeps your appetite low when you've overeaten so you don't gain weight. But fructose distorts this message[28]. That means when you eat fructose, it doesn't add to how many calories your brain has perceived you needed by the end of the day.

Let's go back to the fast food and soda paradox—why can someone go to a fast food joint, have a large soda with fries and a hamburger, but then be hungry enough to eat two or three more times later in the day? A forty-two ounce soda will have approximately 500 to 600 calories, and yet you could refill that once, and still not be full at all from it. You'd still have room for 1,000 more calories from the fries and cheeseburger. Why? What's the difference between calories from the food and calories from the soda? The answer is the soda is sweetened with **pure 100%** high-fructose corn syrup.

As far as your brain was concerned, the soda had no more calories than water. This means that the fructose prevents your brain from perceiving how many calories you: 1) really needed and 2) actually consumed. Your hypothalamus, your internal calorie counter, just missed all those calories. As a result, you overate, gained weight, and only made leptin resistance worse.

When researchers compared a high-fructose diet to a high-glucose one, they found that although the high-fructose diet raised blood sugar less (as expected), it did little to decrease ghrelin, the stomach hormone responsible for the sensation of hunger[32]. The more ghrelin in your gut, the hungrier you feel. The high-fructose diet also produced a far smaller leptin response. The high levels of ghrelin after ingesting fructose are why you still feel enough hunger to eat the hamburger and fries after your large Coke. The lack of leptin is the reason you could eat again a few hours later.

Studies like this bring up an important point. You might find your blood sugar barely rises after drinking a soda, but that doesn't mean the Coke was good for your diabetes, or at least less harmful. Blood sugar is but one part of the metabolic syndrome, and when it comes to high-fructose corn syrup, it is better to eat something healthy that raises blood sugar than to drink a soda! Blood sugar is not always the most important number when it comes to diabetes!

The consumption of HFCS in America has increased more than 1,000% between 1970 and 1990, and HFCS is now used in 40% of the caloric sweeteners added to foods and beverages. It's the sole caloric sweetener in soft drinks in the United States[27].

A very conservative estimate for how much HFCS the average American ingests daily is 132 calories for everyone over two years old. The top 20% of all soda drinkers average 316 calories per day[27]. That's almost an extra 10,000 calories per month that your brain doesn't know you're ingesting. That equates to gaining an extra 2.7 pounds per month, or 33 pounds per year!

The small amount of fructose found in fruit is not going to be a problem for you at all. Have your fill of apples, berries, and melons on the high carb portion. However, beware of fruit juice, soda, baked goods like pastries and doughnuts, and specifically, anything with the words "fructose," "corn syrup," or "high-fructose corn syrup" on the label. Avoid the Eight Cs: candy, cake, cereal, chips, cola, cookies, crackers, & (ice) cream (also white bread, which has enriched flour instead of fructose syrup).

Another problem with taking fructose in large amounts like that found in colas and other sweets is that fructose fills up liver glycogen quickly, a recipe for fat gain. You have two storage spaces for glycogen—a small one in the liver, and a larger one in your muscles. Fructose is stored as glycogen in the liver, and once liver glycogen is full, all other carbohydrates are converted to fat.

This problem can kill your weight loss if you eat the wrong things while carb loading. Basically, after having two large doughnuts in the morning or drinking one or two sodas at lunch, your liver glycogen would be full for the rest of the day. So even if you try to eat cleaner sources of carbohydrates for the rest of the day, those carbohydrates are likely going to just wind up as fat instead of glycogen, the desired storage space.

This sugar found in fruit, juice, soda, and candy fills up liver glycogen very quickly, in as little as one meal. Since fruit in its natural state doesn't contain that much fructose per serving and is very hard to overindulge in, you can and should eat fruit during the carb load. However, no juice, canned fruits, or dried fruits like raisins, dates, or figs! They're so high in fructose that they're nearly as bad for you as a Coke.

> **The worst recipe for fat gain is actually mirrored very closely by millions of Americans daily—ingesting lots of fats and high-fructose corn syrup at the same time.**

Rats fed a diet of 60% fructose for six months who became leptin resistant and then went on to follow a high-fat diet gained nearly twice the amount of fat as those leptin-responsive rats[29]. The worst fat provokers are what many of us do every day, and we need to stop if we're going to put an end to the obesity and diabetes epidemic that is plaguing this country today.

Eating white flour and fat together can be just as damaging. Refined carbohydrates found in white bread, pastries, and croissants will push insulin levels very high, far beyond the appropriate level given the number of carbs in these foods. Food eaten with saturated fat, like in a Big Mac, drives insulin levels even higher. The body preferentially stores refined carbs and saturated fats eaten together as body fat, even if you burn more calories than are in the burger! The good news is that in a depleted state, the carbohydrates in these foods are much more likely to be stored as glycogen than fat. For this reason, you can have a serving or two of an old favorite like pizza or nachos, but not at every meal. More than one cheat meal per day during the carb load is absolutely setting you up for diabetic disaster.

When carb loading, it is critical that you eat clean carbohydrates in proper amounts. Clean carbohydrates are easily defined as carbs void of high-fructose corn syrup and enriched or refined carbohydrates 95% of the time. Save the damage for holidays and other very special occasions.

The Fifth Prescription in Summary

- You need a low-carb diet because you're insulin resistant.
- Even eating a normal amount of healthy carbs can stall weight loss in a diabetic.
- People on low-carb diets burn more calories, feel less hunger, retain more muscle while dieting, and lower their cholesterol and blood pressure.
- A low-carb diet is a high-fat diet. Fats aren't bad, especially the kind you're eating in *The New Diabetes Prescription*.
- Low-carb diets really work because you're instantly removing all fattening foods from your diet 100% of the time.
- Consume four grams of EPA and DHA per day and four tablespoons of flaxseeds.
- Take 50 to 300 mg of 5-HTP and 2,000 mg L-glutamine on the low-carb days if you get sugar cravings.
- If your BMI is over 30, load with clean carbohydrates for one to two days after ten to twelve days of following a low-carb diet. Have about 0.3 grams of carbs per day per pound of body weight.

- If your BMI is under 30, load with clean carbohydrates for one to two days after five days of following a low-carb diet. Have about 0.45 grams of carbs per day per pound of body weight.
- Avoid high-fructose corn syrup, table sugar, and honey.
- Avoid enriched or refined carbohydrates (e.g., candies, colas, cakes, crackers, ice cream, chocolate, cereal, and bread with enriched or refined flour in the label).
- The first two weeks are the hardest, but then it gets easy.
- Use ground flaxseeds, glucomannan powder, psyllium husks, and green vegetables to deal with initial constipation.
- Watch that your blood sugar does not go too low, and speak to your doctor about lowering your medications as necessary.

Now That You Know the Why Of Low-Carb Eating, You Must Learn the What And How

You've learned that a low-carb diet is superior compared to low-fat diets at controlling the various facets of diabetes. You've also learned that you can make it even more effective by including short cycles of eating more carbs, including omega-3s, and taking 5-HTP. Finally, you learned that when you do eat carbs, you must avoid high-fructose corn syrup, refined sugar, and refined flour.

And now it's time to get into the nuts and bolts of the two phases of your diet. The Sixth Prescription will deal with the low-carb part of your diet, including the best proteins, fats, and fibers. The Seventh Prescription will then educate you on how to carb load, including which carbs to choose, which to avoid, and how to bend the rules.

The beauty of this way of eating is that you can have your cake and lose weight too.

You can have a treat every now and then without compromising your health because you made the deliberate choice to eat *this* many carbohydrates at *that* time. That's the agreement you make that gives you the rewards you want. And you have the knowledge that you are in control.

But be warned: insulin resistance can always come back even after you heal. If you go back to your old way of eating, avoid exercise, or gain weight, the metabolic syndrome will come back. Count on it.

Further, if you need a low-carb diet to lose weight, you need a low-carb diet to keep the weight off even when you've reached your weight-loss goals. Increasing your carbs to normal again will put the pounds back on. You need to treat yourself with enough delicious low-carb fare so you can do this for the rest of your life. You're in this for the long haul.

You also can't eat a twenty-ounce prime rib every day and expect to lose weight. You can eat more calories on a low-carb diet and lose weight than on a regular diet, but calories still count! On the bright side, there is now a solution to your disease, a profound and beautiful one, but it will take your effort. And isn't that better than where you are now?

Again, following these prescriptions puts you in control.

SIXTH PRESCRIPTION

Eat the Foods That Heal, Avoid the Foods That Kill

*T*he Sixth Prescription is all about the best and worst choices for all kinds of foods. You will learn about the good, the bad, and the ugly among choices for proteins and fats during the low-carb portion of the diet. You'll also learn the importance of getting enough fiber and water every day.

Don't confuse that message to mean you won't also be including these foods during the carb-loading portion. You will. But you first need to build the foundation of your diet with good fats and proteins, even when you're ingesting carbs alongside them.

It's not enough to just go low carb. You want to fill your body with the highest quality low-carb nutritional sources while avoiding some evil foods like trans-fatty acids that, while they contain zero carbohydrates, can shorten your life nonetheless. Once you determine the best foods to make up your personal diabetic diet, you'll be that much closer to losing the weight, stabilizing your sugar, cholesterol, and blood pressure, and getting off as much medication as possible.

Eating Protein Equals Losing Fat

Losing body fat, not body weight but body fat, is accomplished by building or, at the very least, maintaining muscle mass while coaxing the body to draw on its own fat stores for energy. Anyone who went from 45% body fat to 8% body fat *did that.* Every top fitness book in America seeks to help you achieve that. So it's no wonder that every athlete, actor, actress, and fitness authority all include a portion of protein in each and every one of their meals.

First, dietary protein helps build muscle and prevents it from being used as energy when exercising. Hear me now. You absolutely, positively cannot achieve a large fat loss without including a serving of protein at every meal.

Second, fat loss is about *building* muscles that *get worked* to *burn fat.* The more muscle that's built, the more it can burn. The more muscle you have, the more calories from fat you can burn just sitting around. That's like owning a large business and hiring other people (muscles) to earn (burn) money (calories) for you. I personally burn about 600 more calories per day from twenty-five pounds of extra muscle than if I had never picked up a weight. I burn those calories whether or not I do any exercise that day. Eating protein is the fuel that builds those muscles, but lifting weights is the stimulus.

Third, the act of eating any meal high in protein can raise your metabolism by 25%. Better than that, 30% of the calories you eat from protein at each meal are actually used just to digest it! That means around 10% of the total calories that all those athletes and actors eat in a day are not even being used by the body, but wasted as heat. A 30% boost in your metabolism, by the way, is a better deal than *anything* you can buy in a bottle—unless it reads "methamphetamine" on the front.

> **The act of eating any meal high in protein can raise your metabolism by 25%. Better than that, 30% of the calories you eat from protein at each meal are actually used just to digest it!**

Finally, protein makes you full, and keeps you fuller longer. Protein foods are self-limiting – it's easy to eat a whole box of Girl Scout Cookies, but it's hard to eat a twelve-ounce rib eye. You will voluntarily stop eating food sooner and voluntarily delay your next meal every time you eat a meal high in protein.

Where to Get Your Protein, When, and How Much

The type of protein you eat is as important as the amount you eat. Protein from eggs, cheese, fowl, fish, lamb, pork, beef, low-carb yogurt, and low-carb milk are complete proteins in that they contain all the essential amino acids needed to reap the advantages I've listed above. In contrast, fruit, vegetables, legumes, and grains are incomplete protein sources since they lack one or more of the essential amino acids. Do eat these foods, but *not for the protein!*

Not all protein sources are created equal.

The majority of fitness experts suggest getting about one gram of protein per pound of body weight. I personally get this much, and I agree that it's enough to stimulate muscle growth and give you the benefits described thus far. However, if you're very overweight, this recommendation would have you eating upward of 300 or 400 grams of protein for your 300 or 400 pounds. To call that excessive would be kind to say the least.

If you fall under this category, throw the one gram of protein per pound of body weight rule right out the window. Just get 55 to 60% of your daily calories from fat, and let the rest be protein along with thirty or so grams of carbs.

Be sure to divide the total amount of protein you do consume over five or six meals spread two to three hours apart.

Buy Protein Powders with Whey and Casein

Most of your protein should come from good old-fashioned natural food that was available to your ancestors. Foods like chicken, beef, eggs, fish, and cheese are very slow to digest and take up a lot of space in the stomach compared to protein shakes, making them more likely to keep your blood sugar stable, your stomach full, and your mind free of cravings.

However, there will be times when time is scarce, and you need a source of protein that is faster to prepare than grilled salmon. In fact, there are four times during the day when your body needs a lot of high-quality protein[1-3]: breakfast, right before and during exercise, up to an hour after exercise, and before bed.

Whey protein isolate and micellar casein are the highest-quality proteins you can find in a protein powder. When buying a protein powder, find a mix of these two, or buy one of each. The mixture gives the most bang for your buck in terms of keeping blood sugar stable and repairing muscle after exercise. Look for a brand that has fewer than three carbs per serving like Designer Whey, Isopure, or Metabolic Drive. The best low-carb protein powders are Metabolic Drive, Isopure, Designer Whey, Met-Rx, and BCAAs. Protein bars with whey and casein are also good, so long as they have fewer than five grams of carbohydrate and no high-fructose corn syrup or refined carbs.

Protein Is Not Bad for the Kidneys!

There are still some nutritionists and health care practitioners who have lived under a rock for the last thirty years. I guess there was a convention on medical myths that lasted too long. Nevertheless, some of these people decided nothing has changed in the last thirty years, and still falsely believe the diets with 30 to 40% protein cause kidney damage. There are zero scientific studies to validate this.

> **Eating protein will never cause kidney disease[4], but limiting protein may be a good idea if you already have it[5].**

Because the kidneys play a crucial role in the metabolism of all proteins, a diet with lots of protein may put an extra strain on your already-damaged organ, and not eating extra protein might take the stress off. Excess protein is basically as bad for those with kidney disease as sugar is bad for diabetics. However, the analogy breaks down there since sugar is basically lousy for everyone all of the time, save during and after exercise, whereas protein is healthy for everyone with healthy kidneys all of the time[4]. My own endocrinologist finds nothing wrong with my eating over one gram of protein per pound of body weight, and he is a diabetic himself with kidney disease. The bottom line is that large amounts of protein are OK so long as your kidneys are fine. If they're not, speak with your doctor as to whether you should be limiting protein at one or more meals.

Fat Helps Tremendously with Energy, Blood Sugar, Satiety, and Mood

Fat is far slower to digest than protein or carbohydrates, so when fat is eaten with lower glycemic carbs and proteins, the entire meal is digested far more slowly. This means insulin is released little by little instead of in one giant bolus. The result is less insulin secreted overall, leaving you with more stable blood sugar, longer lasting fullness, increased energy, and fewer cravings.

> **Fat is far slower to digest than protein or carbohydrates, so when fat is eaten with lower glycemic carbs and proteins, the entire meal is digested far more slowly.**

Another part of fat's aid in fullness comes from the greater production of dopamine in the brain. Recall that dopamine is the concentration and energy neurotransmitter. High dopamine levels correlate to feeling alert, focused, and among other factors, *lacking appetite and feeling full after eating.* It would have been difficult for cavemen to fight lions and tigers and bears when all they could think about was nachos and beer, so nature stepped in and gave us this ability to eat in ways that make us hyperalert.

The Facts on Fats

You've probably heard the terms saturated fat, monounsaturated fat, polyunsaturated fat, and hydrogenated fat, also known as trans-fatty acid. However, you may not know that the only difference between all of these types of fats is how many hydrogen atoms they have, and the location of those atoms on the fatty acid.

Fats or fatty acids are organic molecules that do not mix with water. Basically, they look like fish skeletons, as little hydrogen atoms make up the ribs of the carbon spine between a methyl head and a carboxyl tail.

Saturated fats aren't missing any hydrogen atoms at all. They are *saturated* with hydrogen atoms, which is where they get their name. They are solid at room temperature for this reason, and found primarily in butter, coconut and palm oil, and of course animal fat, eggs, and dairy.

Monounsaturated fatty acids (MUFAs) are missing one and only one hydrogen atom. Hence, they are unsaturated by only one hydrogen atom, a.k.a. *mono*unsaturated. The position of the missing hydrogen atom determines the type of monounsaturated fat. They are liquid at room temperature, and found primarily in olive oil, nuts, seeds, and avocados.

Polyunsaturated fatty acids (PUFAs) are missing multiple hydrogen atoms along their chains. Therefore, they are unsaturated many times over, a.k.a. *poly*unsaturated. The positions and number of missing hydrogen atoms determine the type of PUFA. Like

MUFAs, they are liquid at room temperature and found in many of the same foods, specifically canola, safflower, and flax oil, eggs, some fish, some nuts, some seeds, and dark green leafy vegetables.

Trans-fatty acids, also known as hydrogenated acids, are a man-made creation that begins with a PUFA, and replaces the missing hydrogen atoms. Hence this fatty acid has become *hydrogenated*, or transformed, a.k.a. *trans*-fatty acid. The result is a cheap oil that is thicker, can withstand higher temperatures for cooking, and has a longer shelf life. This is the garbage of the fatty acid world, found in commercial cookies, cakes, breads, crackers, but also peanut butter, shortenings, and margarine. The problem is that hydrogenated acids increase LDL (bad cholesterol), increase triglycerides, decrease HDL (good cholesterol), and dramatically raise the risk of heart disease, not to mention they're always found in a food that might as well have been designed to lay fat on your butt and your gut. As of this writing, New York State is trying to pass a law banning them. You'll avoid most of them just by not eating this crap. Do use natural peanut butter and other nut butters over brands with trans-fatty acids on the food label, butter over margarine, and vegetable oils over shortenings.

Saturated Fat Doesn't Necessarily Increase Your Cholesterol!

That saturated fats are bad for you is misleading. First, meats often contain more unsaturated fat than saturated fat. It's just that they even have saturated fat whereas many other foods don't. So they get labeled as bad—but why? While saturated fat can increase LDLs and triglycerides (VLDLs or very low density lipids), cholesterol elevates even more from eating saturated fat and refined carbohydrates at the same time. Recall all the studies previously mentioned that showed low-carb diets lowered cholesterol in diabetics regardless of whether or not they were restricting saturated fat, and that those adding three eggs a day actually improved their good HDL cholesterol.

There is even a certain saturated fat that helps cholesterol levels. Conjugated linoleic acid (CLA) is a saturated fatty acid found in meat, dairy, and cheese that has been shown to increase HDLs, lower LDLs, and increase lean body mass. Supplementing with three grams of CLA per day has been shown to decrease body fat[10] and improve cholesterol, and up to six grams has been shown to add muscle by increasing protein synthesis. However, CLA works best to control body fat levels by avoiding the laying on of fat *when you're overeating*. Basically, more of your gained weight comes on as muscle, and less as fat. How much of a difference can it make? While normal weight gain in the absence of weight lifting is 75% fat and 25% muscle, CLA can help any weight gain level out to 50% fat and 50% muscle[11]! That is worth something!

In *The Fat Flush Plan*, Anne Louis Gittleman mentions a twelve week Norwegian study in which those supplementing with CLA lost 20% body fat with an average weight loss of seven pounds without making any other dietary changes. That is amazing! Think of CLA as an insurance policy against a natural disaster, in this case, weight gain from overindulgence—you'd rather not have it happen, but it's not as devastating if it does. Because it does help with fat loss even when eating normally and it is relatively cheap, I personally take four grams year round.

Finally, We Come to Essential Fatty Acids (EFAs)

The EFAs fall under two different types of polyunsaturated fats, namely omega-3 and omega-6 fatty acids. I've already espoused the essential nature of omega-3s, and how lacking they tend to be in your diet. Omega-6s are found in soybean oil, safflower oil and canola oil. You may also see linoleic acid on food labels, indicating omega-6 fatty acids. While they're essential, you undoubtedly get plenty of them in your diet right now because they are cheaper to use in food than omega-3s, but do not have the same benefits. The average American eats a diet with a ratio around 16:1 of omega-6 to omega-3 fatty acids, when it should be 1:1. Half the battle here is won by dumping processed foods, but the other half is won through direct supplementation from omega-3 rich sources like fish, fish oil, flax oil, and flaxseeds.

The one omega-6 that you should make sure you include in your diet is gamma-linolenic acid (GLA). Like CLA, GLA is another great insurance policy against fat gain, but it takes it a step further. Whereas CLA is most useful for preventing fat gain from overeating, GLA does the same, *plus* it helps you burn fat[14]. Research done at UCLA and UC Berkeley compared supplementing with olive oil or GLA in obese subjects after they lose weight[15]. First, the subjects spent a year losing weight with diet and exercise while taking either 860 mg of GLA or five grams of olive oil per day. For the next two years, the subjects continued to supplement, but received no further dietary advice. After the first year, those supplementing with GLA didn't gain back any weight while the olive oil group gained four pounds. By the second year, the GLA group gained back four pounds, but the olive oil group gained back seventeen! The researchers concluded GLA prevents weight gain by improving insulin sensitivity, impairing body fat creation, and increasing fat burning. GLA is very affordable, and can be found in most health food stores and online at vitacost.com.

My personal preference for EFAs every day is:

- 4,000 mg from a combination of EPA and DHA found in fish or fish oil over two or three meals
- Four tablespoons of milled flaxseeds divided among the last two meals
- Four grams of CLA (although not an EFA) divided into four equal doses
- One gram of GLA divided into three doses

MUFAs and PUFAs should make up the majority of your fats on a low-carb diet. Red meat is OK to eat every day, but EFAs are mandatory to eat every day. You may even have to cut other fats to keep within caloric limit, but it's that important. The Twelfth Prescription will give you a two-week menu that will coordinate every meal and every supplement in the book, including your EFAs, so you can easily see how to put it all together.

Fiber Is the Diabetic Diet's Missing Ingredient

You can do everything right with your nutrition, from avoiding crap sugars and starches, to having less caffeine and more protein. But if you're not getting fiber at every meal, all you're doing is short-changing yourself. You're eating more calories if you're only using food, not fiber, to become full. Studies have shown adding fiber to your diet will improve your blood sugar, blood pressure, and cholesterol[6]. It provides too many advantages for your health and waistline not to be included. Your body was meant to eat meals that includes fibrous foods like fruits, vegetables, nuts, legumes, and seeds.

Fiber comes in soluble and insoluble forms. Soluble fiber found in barley, oats, beans, nuts, barley, apples and oranges, flaxseeds, and psyllium husks is the type of fiber mentioned above that regulates blood sugar and keeps you full. Insoluble fiber like that found in fruits, vegetables, grains, nuts, and seeds helps keep you regular and lowers cholesterol levels[12]. Nearly all foods will contain both, so as long as you focus on including fiber at each meal, you'll be getting plenty from both types.

Adding fiber to any meal, especially one high in carbohydrates, controls glucose in three different ways. First, it basically makes intestinal juice more slippery, making it harder for glucose to pass (slippery little suckers!). Second, fiber binds to glucose, lessening the total amount of sugar in your system that can make an impact. Third, it blunts the actions of amylase, the enzyme responsible for helping digest carbs[7]. The bottom line is that with fiber, less glucose than what you've actually eaten will eventually be absorbed by the body, and over a longer period of time.

As a result, more carbohydrates are used for fuel, and fewer are stored as fat. Fiber is so powerful at this that you can actually use it to blunt the fattening effects of any high-sugar food, should it ever cross your path. Simply taking some flaxseeds or glucomannan along with an ice cream cone *will* reduce some of the fat laid on from that dessert. Most of the carb blockers you see advertised work on this exact principle. Imagine getting that benefit twenty-four hours a day, seven days a week from $2.99 of broccoli over a two-week supply of carb blockers for $19.99.

Fiber adds to satiety by causing the greatest release of cholecystokinin, the "I'm full" hormone, in your stomach. In addition, the slower flow of nutrients out of your stomach keeps you fuller longer. As a result, your blood sugar stays stable and you don't get ravenous at mealtimes. By including it, you wind up eating closer to every three hours instead of every two, and portion sizes remain the same.

Fiber is also a powerful diuretic. Every carbohydrate stored can store three to five grams of water with it, and erratic insulin levels only make it worse. Fiber has been proven to reduce serum insulin levels, which will in turn keep you from gaining excess water. As a result, you'll have less water retention, which may have a favorable impact on your blood pressure.

Adding fiber to your meals will also cause some of the calories from your food to never be absorbed. Instead, they will pass right through your system. Studies show you're probably absorbing around 5% fewer calories per day when getting your twenty-five to thirty-five grams of fiber in your diet[8]. The daily results can be anywhere from 100 to 200 calories for most of the population. That's 54,750 calories saved a year, enough to lose 14.5 pounds without trying!

> **Adding fiber to your meals will also cause some of the calories from your food to never be absorbed. The greatest secret to fat loss is creating a caloric deficit** *without ever knowing it!*

Men should get five to seven grams of fiber per meal and thirty to forty grams of fiber daily. Likewise, women should get four to five grams of fiber per meal for a total of twenty-five to thirty grams. Green leafy vegetables like broccoli, lettuce, asparagus, and cucumbers make a great addition to any meal. Add low-fat dressing to your liking. Eat them plain, cook them, or have them in a salad, just as long as you get your fiber in every meal. When eating carbs, oatmeal with berries or grapefruit will make a terrific way to start the day.

Get the bulk of your fiber from green vegetables by having at least a palm size or more of the veggies at most meals. Some of your fiber can also come from your carb servings. Fruits all have some fiber, grains have less in general, and beans have the most. As previously mentioned, don't count the carbs that are listed under fiber as they aren't treated like carbohydrates by the body.

It is OK to get as many servings of nonstarchy vegetables as you want in a day. You will not be able to binge on them, and your blood sugar will not spike, so they help you to avoid food cravings and fat gain.

Glucomannan, the Best Soluble Fiber on Earth

By far and away, the absolute best form of soluble fiber you should supplement with is glucomannan. In my opinion, it has made psyllium husks obsolete. Glucomannan is the densest soluble fiber on earth, expanding to over 100 times its size when added to water[13]. This property means glucomannan offers the greatest advantage of all four fibers mentioned above!

Once in the stomach, glucomannan's swelling effect will cause all your food to digest much slower. As a result, your digestive system will slow down the rate at which glucose is released. As a result, insulin levels will be lower, making fat loss and energy greater, and appetite less. Cholecystokinin (CCK) will rise while ghrelin falls for hours after ingestion, leaving your hunger nowhere to be found[13].

Having used this product extensively myself, I can tell you firsthand that its ability to bulk up your food and make it heavier has made effortlessly cutting calories without missing them the easiest that it has ever been. For example, I used to make very rich, thick vanilla protein parfaits. Two scoops of vanilla protein powder plus four tablespoons of flaxseeds were needed to reach the correct consistency in the recipe. That comes to 360 calories. I can now reach an even thicker consistency using only one scoop of protein powder and one teaspoon of glucomannan powder, netting 110 calories. No other ingredients are needed—the fiber's ability to expand in water takes care of the rest. This effect is so powerful that I now have to make sure I am not eating too *few* calories per day by including this fiber.

Cassandra Forsythe, author of *The Perfect Body Diet*, suggests adding it to the following foods[13]:

- ***On Low-Carb Days***: cottage or ricotta cheese, creamed vegetables, eggs (salad, scrambled, omelet-style or quiches), ground meats (turkey, salmon, or beef), tuna or chicken salad, smoothies, nut butters, mustard, Greek-style yogurt, and salad dressings

- ***On Carb-Load Days***: low-sugar ketchup or barbeque sauce, gravy, hot whole-grain cereals (oatmeal, oat bran, or cream of wheat), hummus, pesto, soups, tomato sauce, smoothies (with more carbs), salsa, and soy sauce

To get the greatest benefit for fat loss and blood sugar control, men should use ten to fifteen grams of powdered glucomannan per day, and women should use eight to twelve grams. Take the powder in three to four doses over the day for three to five grams for men or two to three grams for women respectively. If you find glucomannan in capsules, break them open and use the powder only. Take glucomannan only as a powder, and never as a capsule - you'll be wasting your money because the powder would just wind up expanding inside the capsule instead of your stomach[13].

Glucomannan tabs can be found online at http://www.vitacost.com, and the powder at http://www.konjacfoods.com. Most health food stores now carry it in some form. You can also search for it under konjac glucomannan.

Drink Half an Ounce of Water
for Every Pound You Weigh

Divide your weight in pounds by two, and get that many ounces of water per day, divided among all but your last meals so you're not getting up to pee all night. Drink sparkling water, lemon water, or even flavored water, avoiding sweetened water if you can. If you insist on drinking sweetened water, make certain it contains an artificial sweetener other than aspartame.

This is the minimum your body needs daily. Water speeds up metabolism by as much as 10% because it is used in nearly every metabolic process in your body. In other words, if you've been de-hydrated for a while, you're not burning as much body fat as you could be. You could be burning only 1,800 calories per day when you should be burning 2,000, and all from not drinking water! That beats many fat burners and costs 0.001% as much!

Soups are so filling because they're mostly water. Vegetables are so filling because they are filled with water, are high in fiber, and low in calories. Some foods are over 90% water, so it really can make a difference in fullness.

A study of obese subjects found that many of them could not distinguish between when they were hungry and when they were thirsty. When they began drinking more water, they naturally lost an average of forty or more pounds over six months because they were no longer confusing the two sensations. Tip: If you're hungry between meals and you know you've eaten enough, try downing two cups of water and see if the sensation goes away within five minutes. If it did, it was thirst, and you haven't been drinking enough. Every time I'm hungry between meals, this works.

Water has also been found to help reduce joint pain, flush tox-ins, increase energy, and even relieve headaches, constipation, and acid indigestion. You're tired when you're dehydrated, and caffeine only makes you more dehydrated. In this way, it is sound advice to drink a glass of water alongside a cup of coffee. The outcome may be more trips to the bathroom, but it will definitely mean increased energy and a faster metabolism in the long run!

The water in coffee, colas, and other caffeinated beverages does not count. Why? Caffeine dehydrates you. The same goes for fat burners, nasal decongestants, antibiotics, and methamphetamines. Even noncaffeinated diet soda does not count. Why? Drink a twelve-ounce can, time when you pee, and roughly how much, and then do the same with twelve ounces of water. You'll pee sooner and more with the diet soda. Again, it dehydrates you.

The Formula for Fullness = Protein + Fiber + Fat - Carbs

You have to create meals that you find delicious and satisfying. Research has validated that the more satisfied you are at your last meal, the less you'll eat at your next[9]. However, satiety in this sense pertains more to how filling the meal was than how well it tasted. In this case, the weight of food is paramount, which is why foods higher in protein, water, and fiber are more satisfying than foods with fewer of these ingredients. Why? Because protein, fiber, and water fill you up without adding a lot of calories. Thirty percent of the protein calories are wasted as heat, and protein also increases stomach hormones that make you full. That is a recipe for fat loss!

If you're particularly hungry at night, especially within two hours before bed, be sure to have a protein snack with almost zero carbs and 30% fat or less. An example would be cottage cheese with flaxseeds or a lean cut of red meat. Never be afraid of having some protein when you're getting carb cravings. If it's between 250 calories of cookies or 250 calories of cheese, you may gain zero fat from the cheese, but that ain't the case with the cookies! Finally, never be afraid of eating extra protein any day you're more active than usual. Hiking, a lot of walking, and an active job all require more calories, and protein is the most metabolically friendly and satiating among the three macronutrients.

The Sixth Prescription in Summary

- Eating protein equals losing fat. Protein increases metabolism, builds and retains muscle, and adds to fullness. Have protein at each meal, once every two to three hours. However, if you have kidney disease, consult with your physician about how much protein you should be getting.

- If buying a protein powder, choose whey-and casein-based ones.

- Fat also adds to fullness and is the fuel your body feeds from on a low-carb diet. The plethora of healthy fats in *The New Diabetes Prescription* will only aid you in your quest for health.

- Saturated fat does not necessarily increase cholesterol, but hydrogenated or trans-fatty acids should be avoided at all times.

- CLA is the best saturated fat and GLA is the best omega-6. Both are terrific fat burners. Have four grams of CLA and one gram of GLA per day.

- The essential omega-3 fatty acids are primarily found in fish, flax, and a few other foods. You want 4,000 mg from EPA and DHA per day, and at least four tablespoons from milled flaxseeds.

- Fiber improves blood sugar, blood pressure, and cholesterol. It also keeps you fuller longer and causes the body to absorb fewer calories from food. Men need thirty to forty grams and women need twenty-five to thirty.

- Drink an ounce of water for every two pounds you weigh.

- The magic feel-full-and-fight-fat meal combo is protein + fiber + fat − carbs. Think salads, salmon and steamed spinach, protein smoothies, nuts and cheese, and eggs in low-carb tortillas.

SEVENTH PRESCRIPTION

Choose Your Carbs Wisely

Carb Loading: Not A Two-Day Junk Food Jamboree

After reading the Sixth Prescription, you're pretty well versed on what foods are appropriate during the low-carb phase of *The New Diabetes Prescription*. In the Seventh Prescription, you'll learn not only the best of all carbohydrate sources to eat, but how to successfully reintroduce old favorites like pizza or ice cream without sabotaging yourself. You'll also learn how to eat goodies during the holidays and other special occasions, and discover extra steps you can take to ensure you don't gain weight.

To be frank, a cyclic carbohydrate diet is *not* a "legal" way to eat crap for thirty-six hours straight.

> **Overeating by a few thousand calories
> of sugar or starch will nullify all the
> other good work you've done.**

What's outlined below will control blood sugar and weight wonderfully if you stay committed to truly monitoring what goes into your mouth. Again, this is not a two day license to binge.

What does that obnoxiously fit man or woman at the party heaping liberal portions of chicken wings, onion rings, and ice cream on their plate know that you don't? That they usually don't eat that way! They don't have great genes, and they're not married to a plastic surgeon (usually). That walking pillar of envy knows that eating *that* much 1% of the time doesn't put a pound on their body in the long term. It was probably the largest cheat meal they had in months, but the rest of the time, they also weren't snacking on celery and ice cubes to look that way. They enjoyed all their other meals, which came from pastures, oceans, and trees—not boxes, cartons, and cans.

> **Habits are what we do most of the time. If we eat well most of the time, we're helping ourselves to stay lean most of the time.**

If we eat something fattening here or there, it only hurts us here or there. By the end of the week, if you've been eating right most of the time, you'll be as lean as you were before you ever laid eyes on that ice cream cake.

> **You must understand that no matter what diet you turn to, you'll wind up eating the exact same types of carbohydrate foods.**

You'll just eat them in different amounts. The most effective diets most commonly used by actors, athletes, fitness enthusiasts, and the men and women who've lost 100, 200, or even 300 pounds are all very similar. They all ate the same carbohydrate foods, and they all avoided the same carbohydrate foods—*habitually*. They all ate apples most of the time, and they all ate pizza every once in a while.

That's the truth, and you need to face it right now. You could run up and down stairs for two hours a day and still gain weight from a junk food diet.

There is no diet for adults without
extraordinarily fast metabolisms that allows
pizza, fries, and milk shakes every day.

Eat Fruits, Vegetables, Legumes, and Whole Grains

Basically, you want to follow the 1,000-Year Rule.

If it wasn't around 1,000 years ago, don't eat it!

There went all frozen dinners, candy bars, sodas, white bread, most pastries, and French fries! You want to eat carbohydrates that are as self-limiting as possible to where you voluntarily stop eating them because your brain and body are telling you that *you have had enough*. That happens when the foods are natural, devoid of refinement or corn syrup, and high in fiber and water. While this list is not complete, each grouping tells you in general how healthy each food is or isn't.

- ***The Best Fruits:*** apples, all berries, cherries, grapefruit, oranges, peaches, pears, plums, and tangerines
- ***Occasionally Acceptable Fruits:*** apricots, grapes, kiwis, mangos, all melons, nectarines, papaya, and pineapples
- ***Diabetically Dangerous Fruits:*** fruit juice, raisins, dates, figs, and all other dried fruits
- ***The Best Vegetables:*** asparagus, broccoli, brussels sprouts, cabbage, cauliflower, celery, cucumber, eggplant, garlic, lettuce, mushrooms, onions, peppers, pumpkin, olives, spinach, tomatoes, turnips, yams, and zucchini
- ***Great Vegetables, but Higher in Carbs:*** beets, carrots, peas, squash, taro, and yucca
- ***Occasionally Acceptable Vegetables:*** baked or

broiled potatoes, corn, tomato juice, tomato soup, and yams

- *Diabetically Dangerous Vegetables*: French fries, mashed potatoes, fried potatoes, hash browns, and creamed soups
- *The Best Legumes:* butter beans, chickpeas, hummus, kidney beans, legumes, lima beans, and navy beans
- *Occasionally Acceptable Legumes*: black-eyed peas, pinto beans, soybeans, unsweetened or artificially sweetened soy milk, and tofu
- *Diabetically Dangerous Legumes:* baked beans, BBQ baked beans, bean dips, refried beans, burritos, chili high in sugar or with refined carbs, bean soups high in sugar or with refined carbs, and any bean cooked with lard or trans fatty acids
- *The Best Whole Grains:* all low-carb grain products, barley, Ezekiel 4:9 products, multigrain bread, oat bran, oatmeal, pumpernickel bread, rye bread, wheat bran, wheat germ, and whole grain bread
- *Occasionally Acceptable Grains:* brown rice, wild rice, amaranth, whole grain bagels, bran flakes, whole grain cereals, whole grain pita, and wheat pasta
- *Diabetically Dangerous Grains:* all cereals high in sugar and refined carbs, corn bread, couscous, sourdough bread, flat bread, white pasta, crackers, white rice, white bread, pastries, cakes, and chips
- *The Best Dairy:* low-carb milk, butter, cream, eggs, cheese, plain Greek yogurt, cottage cheese, and low-carb whey or casein protein powders
- *Occasionally Acceptable Dairy:* plain yogurt, milk, buttermilk, and sour cream

- ***Diabetically Dangerous Dairy:*** canned milk, chocolate milk, milk shakes, yogurt with sugar added, Cool Whip, ice cream, pudding, and milk-based protein powders with more than five grams of carbs per twenty grams of protein

The best carbs listed above are high in fiber and low in calories compared to their size. Therefore, they won't spike blood sugar, keeping your energy high between meals. You'll feel fuller on these foods, so you'll voluntarily eat less. This is why natural foods are so good—it's very difficult to overeat them.

Compare this list to what you're eating now. Dream up some new ideas for quick snacks. Think spinach salad with mushrooms and olives instead of pizza with mushrooms and olives. Think turkey sandwich on whole wheat with fruit instead of cheeseburger with fruit pie. Think cottage cheese with apples instead of apple fritters. These foods are simple, unrefined, and whole. Do you see how different this mindset is from a frozen entrée you pop in a microwave or bag you pick up from a drive through?

A Word on Low-Carb Treats

Refrain from all low-carb ice creams, candies, bars, breads, etc., during the low-carb period. Yes, don't eat the low-carb goodies during the low-carb period. Save them for the high-carb period. They tend to be filled with sugar alcohols that count as carbs no matter what the label reads. They also encourage overeating from other ingredients in the packages. So during the low-carb period, stick to whole foods, and save the snack foods for later. However, protein powder and protein shakes are fine during the low-carb phases.

Your Food Has Factors That Determine How Much It Raises Your Blood Sugar!

You probably know by now that certain foods raise your blood sugar much more than others. The reasons are useful to know so you can develop intuition as to whether a carbohydrate food is going to make you gain fat and get sleepy, or have energy and lose fat:

Acidity: The more acidic a food, the slower it digests. This may seem counterintuitive since you probably know stomach acid is what breaks your food down in the first place. However, extra acid only slows the process down, meaning any foods with vinegar or other natural acids will digest slower than faster. A natural application to this principle is to put lemon juice or anything with lemon or vinegar on your foods. You can also use one to two tablespoons of apple cider vinegar, which is 5% hydrochloric acid, with your meals to lower their glycemic response. Mixed with Stevia in water, it tastes like apple juice.

Amount: A gram of sugar does not raise your blood sugar that much! However, 100 grams will. Always remember that almost any food can be eaten in moderation. It's just that certain foods that lack protein, fiber, fat, and water are not as satiating, and so are a lot easier to overeat on.

Fat Content: This one is tricky. On one hand, the more fat a food has, the slower it digests. Fat is the slowest digesting macronutrient, and carbohydrates are the fastest. So fat can slow the release of carbohydrates out of the digestive system, keeping blood sugar lower. On the other hand, eating the wrong fats with the wrong carbs shoots blood sugar sky high, and insulin with it. The application here is to add fat to high-carb meals, but avoid the killer combination of saturated or hydrogenated fat with HFCS, refined flour, or processed sugar.

Fiber Count: Soluble fiber like that found in glucomannan, oats, beans, nuts, barley, apples and oranges, flaxseeds, and psyllium husks slows down the absorption of all macronutrients and micronutrients in the stomach. Insoluble fiber like that found in fruits, vegetables, grains, nuts, and seeds helps keep you regular and prevents constipation. The obvious application is to get at least five grams of fiber with each meal.

Kind of Starch: Different starches have different molecular configurations, and those different configurations can cause drastic differences in that food's glycemic index. Specifically, rice and potatoes cause your blood sugar to go higher than other starches like oats, wheat, and pasta. The application is to favor oats, whole wheat, and brown pasta over potatoes and white or brown rice as starch choices. Keep this in mind when you read about the Insulin Index below.

Kind of Sugar: Straight glucose raises blood sugar faster than fructose, the fruit sugar. Keep in mind though that while fructose in whole fruit is fine, fructose in soda is terrible because that much of it does not increase leptin.

Physical State: All food is broken down by stomach acid before it is finally used as fuel by the body. Therefore, it makes sense that liquids digest faster than powders, powders digest faster than grains, and grains digest faster than ungrounded solids. The application here is to eat solid foods that are slower to digest for all meals, and if you make protein smoothies, add fiber to them in the form of flax, berries, and glucomannan.

Protein Count: Except for whey protein powder, protein in general is slow to absorb, and will lessen the glycemic effect of the carbs with which it's eaten. Basically, protein lowers blood sugar and increases insulin when combined with carbs[1]. The application here is to always get at least 30% of your calories in a meal from protein to slow the glycemic effect of the carbs in your meal.

Ripeness: Ripe bananas taste sweeter than not fully ripened bananas, and so logically ripe bananas do have a higher glycemic value than unripe ones. In general, ripe fruits have a higher glycemic index than unripe ones. The obvious application here is to eat fruits before they're fully ripened.

Notice that I suggest getting at least 30% of your calories from fat and another 30% from protein on the carb-loading portion. That leaves 40% or less from carbs. The 40/30/30 combination made popular by Barry Sears's *The Zone* is a good example of how to combine types of calories on the weekends.

You Also Have Factors That Determine How Much Food Raises Your Blood Sugar!

Time of Day: Carbs raise blood sugar more in the evening than in the morning because you're more insulin sensitive earlier in the day.

Insulin Sensitivity: The more sensitive your cells are to receiving insulin, the sooner your blood will be cleared of glucose. Moreover, the more insulin sensitive you are, the less likely you will be to store carbs as fat.

Amount of Muscle Mass: The more muscle you have, the more cells you have that need glucose, and the more insulin sensitive you'll be.

Amount and Intensity of Exercise: The longer you exercise the more carbs your body will use. Likewise, the harder you exercise the more carbs you'll process. Sprinting uses more energy than walking, and weight lifting uses more energy than Pilates.

Carb Intake in Relation to Exercise: Carbs are best absorbed during and within one hour after exercise. They are absorbed at this time even better than at breakfast.

Diabetes and PreDiabetes: Type IIs and those with the metabolic syndrome are insulin resistant, and spike higher on carbohydrates since their cells don't receive insulin very well. As a result, sugar stays in the blood, meaning they have *high blood sugar*.

How to Tell If a Food Is Fattening or Fat Fighting

First, is the food in question under the diabetically dangerous categories for carbs? Second, does the food contain any of the following on the label: high-fructose corn syrup, corn syrup, fructose, white sugar, processed sugar, refined flour, white flour, enriched flour? If so, it's fattening and blood sugar spiking! And if it also has saturated or hydrogenated fat, that's the most fattening combination imaginable (remember it's fine to eat saturated fats without carbs like in eggs, meat, or cheese, but never hydrogenated fats). You'll often find these ingredients in baked goods, candy, colas, ice cream, chips, cookies, pizzas, pasta, burgers, and fries.

You should also be wary of savvy food companies who know how to avoid the bad press associated with high-fructose corn syrup. They'll often replace straight sugar and HFCS with less innocuous sounding ingredients like brown rice sugar, maple, agave, cane juice, grape juice, etc. It's all sugar. In fact, agave nectar, a heavily marketed all-natural sweetener, is 90% fructose and 10% glucose[2]. Now, are you ready for the kicker? HFCS itself is only 55% fructose[2]. The rest is glucose. So if HFCS is really bad, imagine how bad agave is. It's amazing this is considered a health food…

Also, be wary of many foods marketed specifically to diabetics. If a nutrition shake in the diabetic section of the drugstore has 20 grams of sugar in it, it's not the best decision for you. For example, Glucerna lists corn maltodextrin and fructose as the first two ingredients after water[3]. One of the most eye-opening experiences of my life occurred the day I suffered a 40 mg/dl hypoglycemic crash from fast-acting insulin while in the hospital. Can you guess what the physician's assistant gave me to get me out of it? Two Glucernas. Of everything she could have given me, that's what she chose. You now know what should and should not be going into your diabetic body. It's time to think for yourself. Don't let companies think for you.

To make sure you're getting the quality you think you are at the grocery store, you'll need to become a label reader. Bread can be brown, but still made with enriched wheat flour or high-fructose corn syrup. Check the ingredients! And if a food still falls under none of the categories above, you should then resort to its glycemic load.

When in Doubt, Base Your Carb Choices on Their Glycemic Load

Ideally, you want to get to the point where you can spot a fattening food from a mile away. For example, I can tell instantly by the texture of bread if it's whole grain or refined, and I'm pretty good at estimating how much butter has gone into various recipes. Still, you're not always going to know beforehand what a food is going to do to your blood sugar and weight. When that happens, the Glycemic Index and Glycemic Load can guide you in the right direction.

Together, they can help you identify over 95% of all carb choices as good, fair, or horrible. They're the science behind why white bread sucks and apples rule. They'll let you determine whether or not a food is OK for you, and how much, for the rest of your life. These indexes give you power, and power gives you freedom.

The Glycemic Index indicates how much blood sugar will rise after eating fifty grams worth of carbohydrates of that food compared to eating fifty grams of carbohydrates from white bread or sugar[4]. It's not surprising that these two foods are used for comparison since they spike blood sugar *really* high. Foods are then separated into highly glycemic, moderately glycemic, or low glycemic on a 0 to 100 scale, 100 being the level to which white bread or table sugar raises your blood sugar.

- High glycemic foods: 55 or greater
- Moderately glycemic foods: between 40 and 55
- Low glycemic foods: below 40

The ideal glycemic level for foods for diabetics is about 50 and below. This includes oats, apples, peaches, pears, all green vegetables, and most beans. The best from the previous list includes mostly low glycemic and a few moderately glycemic carbs in each category. The Glycemic Index of many common foods can be found online at http://www.glycemicindex.com, the official website for the Glycemic Index and Glycemic Database. It has values for almost any food you can think of.

The GI for the most part tells us what we already know. Apples with a GI of 40 are good for fat loss, and doughnuts with a GI[4] of 63 are not. Brown rice is better than white rice because brown rice has a GI of 59 while white rice has a GI[4] of 86. On some scales, white rice is scored even higher.

Unfortunately, the Glycemic Index also has a major limitation. When was the last time you ate fifty grams of carbs from carrots?

Watching a Bugs Bunny marathon? How much is your blood sugar going to rise from ten grams of carbohydrates in carrots? The GI cannot tell you. This is why the concept of the Glycemic Load (GL) was created. It's calculated from the GI and the number of carbs in the food, excluding fiber.

Glycemic Load = Glycemic Index ÷ 100 × [number of carbohydrates − fiber]

- If the GL is less than 10, that food will have a minimal impact on your blood sugar.
- If the GL is between 10 and 20, that food will have a moderate impact on your blood sugar.
- If the GL is greater than 20, that food will have a maximum impact on your blood sugar.

As a diabetic, you want the GL of your meals to be less than 15 when you're eating carbs, and maybe as low as 10. The idea is that meals with total GLs in that range will result in a postprandial blood sugar lower than 140 mg/dl, and ideally no higher than 160 mg/dl.

First example: A slice of rye bread has a GI of 60 and 20 carbs: GL = 60 ÷ 100 × 20 = 12...*not too bad!*

Second example: A white potato has a GI of 100 and 30 carbs: GL = 100 ÷ 100 × 30 = 30...*that's a lot!*

Third example: Two packets of sugar have a GI of 100 and 8 carbs: GL = 100 ÷ 100 × 8 = 8...*not a big deal!*

However, consider this. One of my diabetic friends once spiked her blood sugar from 80 to 180 mg/dl from two packets of sugar on an empty stomach. This is probably due to table sugar's highly processed nature. So if your glucometer reads 180 mg/dl after eating something, whether or not the GL says it should have gone that high, what you ate was too much for you regardless of any number crunching!

Foods That Cause Hypoglycemia

I hate having low blood sugar. I cannot stand eating something sweet, watching my blood sugar swing too high, and then watching it, or even worse feeling it, go too low. I get hungry and tired, and then I overeat.

Many diabetics with still partially functioning pancreases suffer from large blood sugar swings throughout the day. Even without medications that can exasperate this problem like insulin or a sulfonylurea, a diabetic's endogenous supply of insulin can still swing like a pendulum.

Recall from the First Prescription that insulin is excreted in two phases after a meal. The first phase happens within seconds to minutes after the first bite (or even when expecting to take the first bite), and peaks in less than one hour[5]. The second phase is released around the sixty-to ninety-minute mark after the first bite, and peaks one to two hours later. The first, or acute, phase is believed to be far more important in achieving good postprandial blood sugar values hours after the meal, but is also the first bolus affected by type II diabetes[6-7]. If not enough insulin is excreted in the first phase, the body overresponds with insulin in the second phase, and blood sugar can crash.

At other times, the body overresponds to any glucose in the system, using too much insulin for too little glucose. Some researchers say people who do this have "thrifty metabolisms,"[10] because they are trying to store as much glucose away into their muscle and fat cells as possible to save them for the next ice age. Unfortunately, this also turns out to be a pattern for weight gain,[8-9] and occurs the leaner you become or in the earlier stages of the disease. And while there are certain foods that make it worse, there is a tool, the Insulin Index, which helps you find them.

The Insulin Index, the lesser known sibling to the Glycemic Index, is the hypoglycemic's best friend. While the Glycemic Index tells you how much certain foods raise your blood sugar, the Insulin Index measures how hard it is to bring that blood sugar back down after it has gone up.[11-12] Like the Glycemic Index, the Insulin Index is also measured on a scale from 0 to 100, the highest value being assigned to white bread for comparison's sake. Then foods are measured first to see how much they raise blood sugar (Glycemic Index) and cause the release of insulin compared to white bread (Insulin Index).

Most foods cause your postprandial (after eating) blood sugar to rise about as much as they cause it to fall[11]. They have relatively the same Glycemic and Insulin Index values. For example, corn flakes have a Glycemic Index of 76 and an Insulin Index of 75, meaning they raise your blood sugar 76% as much as straight white bread, and lower your blood sugar 75% as much as white bread. Apples have a Glycemic Index of 50 and an Insulin Index of 59, meaning they raise your blood sugar about 50% as much as white bread, and lower your blood sugar 59% as much as white bread. So far, it seems blood sugar is moving in tandem with insulin. All foods that raise your blood sugar to a certain level come down at the same rate, and to around the same level. *But that is not always the case.* What happens when we test processed starches and sugars?

Researchers discovered these foods caused your blood sugar to rise more than they caused it to later fall[11]. They all had a substantially higher Glycemic Index than Insulin Index. For example, brown rice was found to have a GI of 104, but an II of 62, and white rice had a GI of 110 but an II of 79! Rice then is statistically likely to keep your blood sugar high for a very long time. This adds to why rice is *not* a good choice for weight loss. Anecdotally, five different diabetics (a type I and four type II's) all rated white rice as the greatest blood sugar "spiker" of any food they'd ever encountered.

Another minority of foods caused your blood sugar to drop more than they caused it to rise in the next few hours[11]. These foods have a substantially higher Insulin Index than Glycemic Index. Yogurt has a Glycemic Index of 62 but an Insulin Index of 115! Statistically, your blood sugar is likely to be lower ninety minutes after eating yogurt than right before eating it! However, other than yogurt, every other food in this category *was high in refined carbs and high-*

fructose corn syrup. Again, you won't get full and stay full on these foods. The Insulin Index therefore can be used by diabetics and hypoglycemics to cut back on highs and lows, keep energy higher, and minimize cravings.

Before I knew about the Insulin Index, I used to use nonfat plain yogurt with some protein powder and fiber to raise my blood sugar before I worked out on my carb-loading days. But within forty-five minutes of eating, my blood sugar would be in the 60s – the low end of normal! No one feels like working out at that level, and people don't usually get that low. Then once I started exercising, my blood sugar routinely went into the 40s and 50s, and these values are where it gets dangerous.

After I learned that yogurt typically causes blood sugar to drop more than it causes it to rise, I wondered if that was the cause of my lows. I immediately tried rice milk, made solely from white rice, since it causes blood sugar to rise more than it caused blood sugar to fall according to the Insulin Index. Remember that during and after exercise are the best times to take in high GI foods.

Lo and behold, my typical preworkout blood sugar went from an average of 65 mg/dl to an average of 105 mg/dl. *And all I did was have fifteen grams of sugar from white rice instead of yogurt.* When I told this to one diabetes researcher, she shook her head in amazement and said, "The things we don't even know that we don't even know..."

The Insulin Index is fairly new. There are not that many tested foods as of now that show a disproportion between glycemic rise and insulin rise (glycemic fall). However, many studies on the insulin effects of refined carbs have shown these foods provoke out-of-this-world insulin levels. It's safe to assume foods with these ingredients will behave like cake and cookies did below. Here are some foods that show at least a 15% discrepancy in insulin score above or below the glycemic score[12]:

Foods That Crashed Blood Sugar		
Food	**Glycemic Score**	**Insulin Score**
Cake	56	82
Yogurt	62	115
Ice cream	70	89
Cookies	74	92
Mars bar	79	112
Jelly beans	118	160
Foods That Spiked Blood Sugar		
Food	**Glycemic Score**	**Insulin Score**
All-Bran	40	32
Oatmeal	60	40
Muesli	60	40
Brown pasta	68	40
Brown rice	104	62
White rice	110	79
Crackers	118	87

The lesson here is simple. If you lose a lot of weight, or are in the earlier stages of diabetes, you're going to be in my shoes, and find that your blood sugar may swing high and low on your carb-load days. And after it swings low after a huge bolus of insulin, you're going to be hungry again and prone to overeating. Even on your low-carb days, getting all of your carbs in one sitting from something highly glycemic is bound to jump-start your cravings. So pay attention to your appetite in response to carbs as you lose weight.

Personally, I've discovered that eating lots of fruit and honey on my high-carb weekends leads to weight gain, and restricting fruit to berries, cutting honey, and adding some starches leads to weight loss. My appetite is also much better. I can get so hungry so fast from eating a little fruit, cottage cheese, and toast with honey, but so full from having crepes made from whole wheat with berries. Sprinkling starchy, low glycemic Ezekiel cereal on Greek yogurt, low in carbs and high in protein, fills me up for hours.

Also, no matter what these indexes tell you, garbage is still garbage. For example, as you read, HFCS does not raise blood sugar that much, but it is still awful. Never use these indexes to justify a food as less crappy than you'd like to believe. Keep your carb choices below a GI of 50 on your carb days, be moderate in your use of carbs to maintain a low GL, and be wary of foods with a much higher or lower II than their GI; there are only a handful of these right now, but more surprises will come up as more research comes out.

Eating Old Favorites on the Weekends: Have Your Cake and Lose Weight Too

It is very difficult to tell someone to *never* do something again. Recovering alcoholics are usually advised to quit drinking forever, and that fact juxtaposed against their addiction is what makes abstaining so hard. Fortunately, a few chocolates have, to my knowledge, never caused anyone to cause a high-speed accident or drive a man to beat his wife and children. These two facts make it OK for you to have your favorite temptations from time to time. But there is a catch. You have to decide in advance how much you're going to have, and how often you're going to have it.

Two slices of pizza can't turn into four, no matter how much your friends are eating. Be social by talking to them—they chew, you talk. One scoop of ice cream can't become three no matter how insistent your date or friend is. At that moment in time, you have to say "no," and you have to say "I've had enough," and you have to stick to that. However, the only way you can say those words is if you know *how much enough is*.

I'll put it to you this way. If drinking is your thing, you can't have New Year's Eve once a week, and if eating is your thing, you can't have Thanksgiving once a week. In reality, to stay lean for life, you can only have New Year's Eve on December 31 and Thanksgiving on the third Thursday in November. For the rest of the year, you can have two drinks on one day and a burger and fries on another.

> **How do you know how much of a food you should eat, or if you should even eat any of that food? It's simple. If you can answer with a specific amount that does not leave you stuffed, rolling away from the table in a food coma, it's probably OK to eat. However, if the answer is "there is never enough," then the only answer you should give is "none at all."**

I get into trouble with this question with ice cream cake. Ask me how much mud pie is "enough," and I'll probably tell you the whole cake. It is a hard fact that I once ate half an ice cream cake, a protein shake, and several cookies after a bad insulin overdose years ago. Even the common occurrence of an ice cream cake in the kitchen and a stressful day at work can throw me over the edge. For me, one slice of mud pie does not suffice. Ten might. That is the difference between addiction and indulgence. Alcoholics will always answer "there is never enough" to alcohol, which is why they have to abstain for life. I can answer that same question with "one shot of Grey Goose," and that is why I may partake. You may say "three pancakes are enough," but I say "eight with butter, syrup, and whipped cream," which is why I abstain.

To summarize, before you can decide on how much, on what, and when to indulge, you must answer three questions. Are you able to voluntarily decide on a stopping point that leaves you satisfied? Is the only amount that leaves you satisfied too much? Can you keep your word in an environment that you do not control, like at a party or with a pushy friend?

Surviving the Holidays and Other Special Occasions with Your Waistline Intact

As Clarence Bass (http://www.cbass.com), a man who is leaner at more than seventy years old than most gymnasts at twenty, has said, "No one ever got fat in one day." It's true. A day of overeating on the holidays is not what leads to obesity in America. However, days and days of overeating around the holidays certainly will. Halloween, Thanksgiving, Christmas, and New Year's are four days over a span of sixty-two days. That leaves fifty-eight days between them to lose fat. But that doesn't happen because of leftovers, gift baskets, and get-togethers.

The solution is so simple. Eat big for one day, but be done at bedtime. Don't eat big for a week, and certainly not for an entire season. Leftovers will be left over around your middle if you keep them around. Therefore, get rid of *all* of your leftovers, or make far less food. Feel guilty? Give those foods away. Give it to the homeless. Give it to your guests in packages to take home. But get the leftovers out of your house. I don't know of one fitness expert who does not believe in the adage that you will eventually eat any food in your home. If it's there, it will eventually be eaten. So just get rid of it.

For example, not that I recommend you eat this much, but check out the menu on the next page. Now, suppose you were planning on having *that* on Thanksgiving.

A Typical Thanksgiving Feast

Food	Amount	Fat	Protein	Carbs	Fiber	Calories
Turkey	6 Ounces	24	47	0	0	404
Gravy	1/2 Cup	2	2	6	0	50
Stuffing	1 Cup	18	6	38	6	338
Buttered Croissants	2 pieces	24	10	50	2	456
Pecan Pie	1/8 Piece	27	6	64	0	523
Pumpkin Pie	2 Slices	13	5	44	2	313
Mashed Potatoes	1 Cup	9	4	32	3	225
Coffee	2 Cups	8	1	2	0	84
Red Wine	2 Glasses	0	0	4	0	150
		125	81	240	13	2,543

That's a recipe for fat gain and high blood sugar. How could you step up your exercise and cut your calories ever so slightly so you wouldn't gain a pound during that week? Simple. First, you'd eat the following foods and take the following supplements. You'll find an explanation for all the supplements in the Ninth Prescription and the recipes in the Tenth Prescription.

How to Lose Fat During the Holidays

Drink Green Tea 5 Times A Day Every Day

	Saturday & Sunday	Monday - Wednesday	Thanksgiving	Friday - Monday	Tuesday – Friday
Meal 1	Breakfast Burritos: 8 Carbs & 240 Calories	Cheese Omelet: 3 Carbs & 370 Calories	Cheese Omelet: 3 Carbs & 370 Calories	Cheese Omelet: 3 Carbs & 370 Calories	Cheese Omelet: 3 Carbs & 370 Calories
30 min. before	1,000 mg Taurine	1,000 mg Taurine	1,000 mg Taurine	1,000 mg Taurine	1,000 mg Taurine
	300 mg Pantethine	300 mg Pantethine	300 mg Pantethine	300 mg Pantethine	300 mg Pantethine
	Multivitamin	Multivitamin	Multivitamin	Multivitamin	Multivitamin
As needed	Vitamin C	Vitamin C	Vitamin C	Vitamin C	Vitamin C
Meal 2	NDP Mocha Super Shake: 5 Carbs & 290 Calories	NDP Vanilla Super Shake: 2 Carbs & 240 Calories	NDP Vanilla Super Shake: 2 Carbs & 240 Calories	NDP Vanilla Super Shake: 2 Carbs & 240 Calories	NDP Pumpkin Super Shake: 4 Carbs & 250 Calories
2 each	CLA & GLA	CLA & GLA	CLA & GLA	CLA & GLA	CLA & GLA
	2,000 mg Carnitine	2,000 mg Carnitine	2,000 mg Carnitine	2,000 mg Carnitine	2,000 mg Carnitine
	100 mg CoQ10	100 mg CoQ10	100 mg CoQ10	100 mg CoQ10	100 mg CoQ10
Alpha Lipoic Acid	300 mg ALA	300 mg ALA	300 mg ALA	300 mg ALA	300 mg ALA
Meal 3	Chicken Caesar Salad with 2 tbls. low-carb Caesar Dressing: 3 Carbs & 310 Calories	Chef Salad with Regular Italian Dressing: 3 Carbs & 310 Calories	Lox & Cream Cheese: 1 Carbs & 200 Calories	Chef Salad with Regular Italian Dressing: 3 Carbs & 310 Calories	Spinach Salad with 2 tbls. low-carb Greek Dressing: 3 Carbs & 350 Calories
30 min. before	1,000 mg Taurine	1,000 mg Taurine	1,000 mg Taurine	1,000 mg Taurine	1,000 mg Taurine
	300 mg Pantethine	300 mg Pantethine	300 mg Pantethine	300 mg Pantethine	300 mg Pantethine
	15 mg Biotin	15 mg Biotin	15 mg Biotin	15 mg Biotin	15 mg Biotin
	4,000 IU Vit. D	4,000 IU Vit. D	4,000 IU Vit. D	4,000 IU Vit. D	4,000 IU Vit. D
Meal 4	NDP Mocha Super Shake: 5 Carbs & 290 Calories	NDP Vanilla Super Shake: 2 Carbs & 240 Calories	Thanksgiving Dinner: 240 Carbs & 2,540 Calories	NDP Vanilla Super Shake: 2 Carbs & 240 Calories	NDP Pumpkin Super Shake: 4 Carbs & 250 Calories
2 each	CLA & GLA	CLA & GLA	CLA & GLA	CLA & GLA	CLA & GLA
	2,000 mg Carnitine	2,000 mg Carnitine	2,000 mg Carnitine	2,000 mg Carnitine	2,000 mg Carnitine
	100 mg CoQ10	100 mg CoQ10	100 mg CoQ10	100 mg CoQ10	100 mg CoQ10
Alpha Lipoic Acid	300 mg ALA	300 mg ALA	300 mg ALA	300 mg ALA	300 mg ALA

How to Lose Fat During the Holidays

Drink Green Tea 5 Times a Day Every Day

	Saturday & Sunday	Monday - Wednesday	Thanksgiving	Friday - Monday	Tuesday – Friday
Meal 5	2 Servings Orange Roughy with Salsa: 8 Carbs & 240 Calories	Vanilla Shake: 4 Carbs & 190 Calories	Have Nothing	Vanilla Shake: 4 Carbs & 190 Calories	Low-Carb Pizza: 3 Carbs & 270 Calories
	1,000 mg Taurine	1,000 mg Taurine	1,000 mg Taurine	1,000 mg Taurine	1,000 mg Taurine
	300 mg Pantethine	300 mg Pantethine	300 mg Pantethine	300 mg Pantethine	300 mg Pantethine
	1,500 mg Inositol	1,500 mg Inositol	1,500 mg Inositol	1,500 mg Inositol	1,500 mg Inositol
4 billion cells	Beneficial Bacteria*	Beneficial Bacteria*	Beneficial Bacteria*	Beneficial Bacteria*	Beneficial Bacteria*
Meal 6	Lox & Cream Cheese: 1 Carb & 200 Calories	Have Nothing	Have Nothing	Have Nothing	Chocolate Shake: 7 Carbs & 210 Calories
	1,000 mg Magnesium	1,000 mg Magnesium	1,000 mg Magnesium	1,000 mg Magnesium	1,000 mg Magnesium
	200 mg B6	200 mg B6	200 mg B6	200 mg B6	200 mg B6
60 min before bed. Double if needed.	0.5 mg Melatonin	0.5 mg Melatonin	0.5 mg Melatonin	0.5 mg Melatonin	0.5 mg Melatonin
	100 mg 5-HTP	100 mg 5-HTP	100 mg 5-HTP	100 mg 5-HTP	100 mg 5-HTP
	100 mg Theanine	100 mg Theanine	100 mg Theanine	100 mg Theanine	100 mg Theanine
Calories	1,570	1,350	3,350	1,350	1,700
Carbs	30	14	246	14	24

* Please see multivitamin, vitamin D, and probiotics under the Ninth
Prescription for a description of beneficial bacteria and their benefits.

The calories on each day above (except Thanksgiving) are appropriate for someone who burns 1,600 to 1,800 calories per day. I've cut calories by around 20% for three days prior and three days after Thanksgiving to create enough of a caloric deficit to mitigate any damage done on Turkey Day. That's it. The strategy here is to burn enough fat to make room for the fat gain. If you burned 1,700 calories per day, you'd be leaner on the Tuesday after Thanksgiving than you were the previous Saturday by following the above. The supplements further help lower your blood sugar while boosting your metabolism. And while this alone would counteract the gluttony, stepping up the exercise only makes it more effective.

You'll step up exercise four days before and up to four days after the big day, utilizing brief, intense cardio. Sprinting, jumping rope, elliptical trainers, and kettlebells are all wonderful exercise choices. For example, this simple, repetitive, and highly effective program would do well:

1) Warm-up with mobility drills for five minutes.
2) Do swings for twenty to thirty seconds, rest twenty to thirty seconds, and repeat ten to fifteen times.
3) Go for a walk to cool down for as little as five minutes to as long as you like.
4) Stretch your hips for five minutes.

In as little as twenty minutes a day, you can have all your exercise done, and not gain a pound over the holidays. It's really not that hard.

> **During any special occasion where you *plan in advance* to eat big, you should also exercise intensely as close to eating time as possible. Fifteen minutes of extremely high-intensity exercise done before you get ready for the night will keep your metabolism elevated 10-15%, and can triple your body's tolerance to high-carb foods. Your body will want those carbs, and use them for fuel like an athlete's body.**

For that reason, you'll want to plan your exercise on Thanksgiving a few hours before you eat. You undoubtedly will have responsibilities like entertaining guests, driving to someone's home, cooking, or making last-minute grocery runs, or all four, but you also have to shower. So before you shower, do that HIIT in your bedroom, garage, outside, or wherever else you choose. Then shower, and go on with your life. In addition, you can also exercise after the meal (if you can roll away from the table). Forty-five to sixty minutes on an elliptical trainer can burn hundreds of calories. How do you know if you should? Because since you planned it, you'll know the caloric cost of food. Just like knowing how much money you have in your bank account, you're going to know how many calories you have to spend.

Also, understand a calorie is not a calorie – a six-ounce chicken breast has 250 calories from protein and fat, and may induce fat loss. A candy bar also has 250 calories, but from sugar and fat. Whatever treat you finally decide on, have your carbs with some fat, fiber, and protein to slow the release of sugar into your system, feel fuller[13-14], minimize insulin release, and further blunt fat gain. Fibers like glucomannan can block or slow the absorption of carbohydrates, ensuring they pass through the system unused. Likewise, have your alcoholic and caffeinated beverages with food to lessen any hypoglycemia.

Finally, pay attention to your appetite following the big days of overeating. With the food out of the house, temptation will be drastically removed, and you'll notice you're actually not that hungry. Cue in on this – it's leptin at work in your favor. Your metabolism is running faster and your appetite is suppressed. This is another reason why we cut calories after the big day. For the three to five days after, feel free to cut back on total calories, cut carbs to below twenty grams per day, but do continue to get at least one gram of protein per pound of body weight. Within ten days, you'll have lost all of the fat, and then some since you're going to be exercising. With the right habits, you can enjoy your holidays, but not pay so damn much for them. Won't that be nice?

How to Handle Alcohol

The rule here is simple. Have no more than two alcoholic drinks over the weekend, none on the weekdays, and count mixed drinks like margaritas and Bloody Marys as two drinks.

Alcohol may have health benefits, but in terms of fat loss, alcohol is an enemy. It's the one substance worse than a fried Twinkie in terms of fat loss. It may be good for the heart, and it may someday be found "to lower the chance of abdominal cancer by 15% in clinical trials," but it will still be an enemy of fat loss.

Drink alcohol because you like the taste, but don't confuse it for a health food. Exercise is good for your heart and your waistline. Alcohol is marginally good only for your heart – and only if it's red wine, so it's not the alcohol that's beneficial. Any pounds gained from drinking it would only make exercise harder, which would negatively impact your heart. That's a study that hasn't been done yet!

Alcohol has seven calories for every gram, meaning one shot of your favorite spirit has 80 to 100 calories. A beer has 150 calories, and the average margarita has 350 calories[15]. However, unlike the fried Twinkie, alcohol doesn't even have a chance of being used for energy. It goes straight to fat. It does nothing else. For the entire time that your liver is metabolizing alcohol, fat burning is shut down.

On top of that, alcohol causes a cascade of negative metabolic reactions. First, alcohol impedes hepatic glycogen production, the effect being increased carb cravings as your blood sugar goes low. Second, alcohol increases leptin and insulin resistance. These are the long-term ways your body reprograms itself to store fat and lower metabolism. It does everything a lifetime of eating refined carbs and sugar can do, but in much less time.

Alcohol also lowers testosterone levels and wastes muscle. Body fat will rise and muscle will waste away. Why the American Diabetes Association's recommended allotment is two drinks a day is beyond me. If you really want to get control of your blood sugar and weight, you'll ignore that advice.

But let's cut to the chase. One four-ounce shot of vodka in some diet Sprite is about 100 calories. That's nothing. Anyone can have *one* of those per week and lose weight. Some could have three. Even 1,000 calories of alcohol per week could be burned off. It's possible on paper. So why is losing weight when drinking such an abysmal failure in practice?

Beyond the metabolic damage done, binge drinking *does not* put you in the mental or physical state to get out of bed bright and early the next morning, start the day with a healthy breakfast, and later exercise. The effects of alcohol on healthy eating and exercise go far beyond the time spent drinking. Read that again. The effects of alcohol on healthy eating and exercise go far beyond the time spent drinking.

Just consider the mental state of someone who drinks heavily even once per week. You've just gone completely out of control for several hours. Are you now going to just switch to a state of complete moderation in eating and exercise for the rest of the week? You can't. You can't be both people.

After heavy drinking with your blood sugar and neurotransmitters tanked, your cravings for salt, fat, and sugar will be through the roof. You will *not* feel like cottage cheese for breakfast. You will *not* feel like going to the gym. You *will* feel like burritos, ice cream, and sitting around all day. You do not trade five hours at a bar for five hours of your life. You lost that five and twenty-five after. That's thirty hours of fat gain.

Drinking requires moderation in order to lose weight. If you and your friends spend every Friday and Saturday night drinking, your friends are actually going to have to get used to you not being that person anymore. You will have to trade being that person for being leaner.

Alcohol has no place during the weekday low-carb phase. Save it for the weekend, and keep it to one drink or two beers for every 100 pounds of body weight per day. That's all you need.

Enough Already—What the Hell Do I Eat?

By far and away, your biggest challenge is coming up with what to eat at work, for dinner, on the road, and at parties. There are a million choices, but right now, you can probably think of only five. This will change. Check out the recipes in the Tenth Prescription, get a low-carb cookbook, search for low-carb recipes online, and learn to adapt your favorite recipes to the low-carb lifestyle. Again, the Twelfth Prescription will help you organize your meals and offer a start-up diet. There are low-carb versions of every food you can think of. It is simply a matter of adapting recipes, and not one of prolonged deprivation.

You can learn more about the caloric and carbohydrate content of foods by going to http://www.nutritiondata.com. This is a wonderful site that gives the complete macro- and micronutrient breakdown of every food, its glycemic load based on different serving sizes, and then some. It is my top unsolicited recommendation for information on the internet.

The Seventh Prescription in Summary

- Carb loading is not a license to binge. Eating carbs on the weekends boosts metabolism, improves insulin sensitivity, and reduces carb cravings. Food is fuel.
- The best carb choices are fruits, vegetables, legumes, and whole grains found in their natural state. In other words, fruits are not turned to jam, vegetables are not turned into syrup to sweeten soda, legumes are not fried, battered, and served with ketchup, and whole grains are not refined into white bread.
- Refrain from all low-carb ice creams, candies, bars, breads, etc., during the low-carb period. Protein powders and shakes are fine anytime.
- The main factors in food that determine how much a carb raises your blood sugar include its acidity, amount, fat content, fiber content, protein content,

type of starch or sugar, physical state, and ripeness.

- The main factors in you that determine how much a carb raises your blood sugar include the time of the day when you eat them, your insulin sensitivity, your total muscle mass, how much and how intensely you exercise, how closely you time eating your carbs to the time you exercise, and of course, whether you already are diabetic or prediabetic.

- Avoid the carbs under the diabetically dangerous categories above, and ensure none of the following are on the food label: high-fructose corn syrup, corn syrup, fructose, white sugar, processed sugar, refined flour, white flour, or enriched flour.

- The Glycemic Index tells you how much 50 grams of carbohydrate in a certain food raise your blood sugar compared to 50 grams of carbs from white bread or sugar. Search for glycemic carbs lower than 40 at http://www.glycemicindex.com.

- The Glycemic Load tells you how much of any amount of a given food will raise your blood sugar. You want to eat meals with a Glycemic Load lower than 15.

- The Insulin Index tells you how much a food will raise your insulin levels. Avoid the refined and processed foods to stay out of the extreme ranges of the Insulin Index.

- Choose the foods you indulge in carefully, and plan those indulgences in advance. You have to know how much is enough before you start eating, and you have to stop once you've had that amount.

- Have no more than two alcoholic drinks over the weekend, none on the weekdays, and count mixed drinks like margaritas and Bloody Marys as two drinks.

It's Time to Talk Calories

In the last two Prescriptions, you've learned how to create a low-carb diet with periodic carb cycles. You've also learned the best foods from which to build the ultimate diabetic diet. However, you still don't know how much fuel is appropriate for your new life. The next Prescription will teach you all about calories. Once you have this next piece of the puzzle, you will know the nuts and bolts of your new lifestyle. All that remains will be finding recipes, deciding on meals, and heading to the grocery store. We'll explore that idea in the Twelfth Prescription.

EIGHTH PRESCRIPTION

Know What, When, and How Much to Eat

*M*any people believe weight loss on a low-carb diet means just that – eat anything and everything so long as it's very low in carbohydrates. Unfortunately, this is simply not true. You can't make lasting changes to your health eating nothing but bacon and cream cheese. The quality of food matters just as much as how many carbs and how many calories.

> **Many people also believe how much weight you gain or lose depends on how many calories you eat. That's also technically incorrect. It's not how many calories you eat—it's how many you absorb. What you eat, when you eat it, and how much you eat all change how many calories you burn daily.**

It's absolutely true that you have to overeat by 3,500 calories to gain a pound of fat. However, it is absolutely false that you gain that weight for every 3,500 extra calories you *eat*. Instead, you gain weight for every 3,500 *extra* calories you don't waste as heat, burn for fuel, or store as glycogen!

Why Naturally Lean People Have a Caloric Advantage

When a calorie enters your system, it is subjected to one of five fates. It can be synthesized as muscle, fat, or glycogen, burned off, or completely wasted as heat. The average person wastes 10% of their fat calories, 10% of their carbohydrate calories, and a whopping 30% of their protein calories as heat. Naturally thin people waste a lot of their calories by expelling them as heat, and naturally heavier people are extremely efficient with their calories, wasting almost none of them. Likewise, a type II diabetic or anyone who's been heavy all her life may be using almost 100% of her carbohydrate calories without any release of fat. Sucks, doesn't it?

The solution to weight loss then is to maximize how many calories you burn per day, how many calories come from *fat*, and to decrease appetite while increasing satisfaction from food. To learn those strategies is the purpose of this Prescription.

Eat Five To Six Times a Day, Every Two to Three Hours, Making Breakfast Your Largest Meal

You won't find a weight-loss book, fitness guru, actor, or professional athlete who does not divide their meals this way. The division of meals from two to three to five to six sets your metabolism up for success for the rest of the day. Most people favor large dinners over large breakfasts, so it is vital that you understand just how important having a smaller dinner and eating five to six smaller meals is. Not having time is an unacceptable excuse – there are surgeons with other people's lives literally in their hands who do this, so do you really want to tell me you can't? You can. I have for ten years in a thousand different environments. You had better be on the moon or in combat if you think you can excuse yourself from eating every three hours.

Our metabolisms run faster when we eat frequent small meals instead of sporadic ones. Digestion is one major way your body burns calories, so the very act of digesting food six times a day instead of two or three is responsible for causing your body to burn an extra 10% to 15% more calories.

Eating frequent small meals also makes you eat fewer calories by the end of the day. Research has confirmed that if I give you one-third of your daily calories for breakfast at 6 AM, or feed you that same number calories divided into six mini-meals at 6, 7, 8, 9, 10, and 11 AM, you'll eat 25% more calories for lunch eating the one big breakfast.[19] One reason may be that both insulin and glucose boluses (increases) are far smaller in frequent small meals, making for more stable blood sugar and a more stable appetite.

Frequent small meals control appetite and blood sugar better than larger, less frequent ones. In fact, cholesterol, glucose, insulin, and even cortisol levels are all lower when eating little by little over the day.

This was verified by feeding subjects seventeen snacks or three large meals per day[20]. Studies of people who eat the most either at breakfast or dinner always show breakfast eaters losing more body fat at the same caloric and activity level. That means if you and your twin both ate 1,500 calories a day, but you ate the most at night while your twin ate the most in the morning, your twin would wind up losing much more weight from fat than you! This is probably because eating breakfast versus skipping the meal will raise your metabolism by as much as 20%.

Unless you exercise in the evening, you burn the most calories in the morning and the least at night. So you should eat the most calories in the morning and eat the least at night.

On your high-carb days, it is better for you to eat your highest-carb meals in the morning and go low carb at night because you are the most insulin sensitive in the morning[23]. Subjects given large amounts of glucose in the morning and later at night had 50% higher blood sugar levels in the evening, but the same amount of insulin, indicating insulin resistance was to blame for the higher blood sugar levels[24]. The reason is because your muscles are less glucose sensitive later in the day. This might not make a difference if you decide to eat clean all day, but it is definitely better for you to have pizza for lunch instead of dinner! You'll likely process those calories better the earlier you eat them.

If you do skip breakfast, you'll be ravenous by 10 AM. Recall that cortisone's first famous dip happens around this time. This is when you'll find yourself running for sugar and caffeine. Lunch and dinner will also wind up being huge, which is only going to cause fat gain. This is the pattern that creates those evening munchies! If you do find you get into trouble with overeating at night, you're not the only one. Researchers even discovered healthy college students did not feel as full and satisfied with their evening meals compared to their earlier ones[22].

> **You tell me if you're going to be able to fend off overeating at night if you skimp on food during the day. A few morning snacks of eggs or cottage cheese are all that's necessary to change your life. People have spent more time deciding which movie to rent.**

Ways Your Body Burns More Calories

- Eating more in the AM than the PM.
- Having a small meal now "to save" for a big meal later.
- Eating more calories from protein.
- Performing brief intense exercise instead of long easy exercise.
- Eating protein at every meal.

- Eating a high-protein meal compared to a calorically equivalent high-carb meal.
- Eating the bulk of your carbs for breakfast, during exercise, and after exercise.
- Eating six small meals instead of three larger ones with equal calories.
- Eating more fats rich in omega-3s like flaxseeds, walnuts, fish oil, salmon, and other fresh water fish, plus GLA and CLA.
- Drinking green tea with each meal.
- Drinking oolong, white, or yerba maté tea with each meal.
- Eating more raw fruits and vegetables.
- Cycling your calories slightly up and down week by week.

Ways Your Body Burns Fewer Calories

- Skipping a meal.
- Skipping a meal "to save" for a big meal hours from now.
- Having cola, white bread, and sugar in your diet.
- Losing sleep.
- Eating more calories from refined sugar and carbs.
- Not getting enough fiber.
- Eating the bulk of your carbs at night.
- Eating fats and carbs together in a meal containing fewer than 30% of the calories from protein.
- Not drinking enough water.
- Drinking alcohol (while red wine might be good for the heart, it is absolutely not good for the waistline).
- Yo-yo and crash dieting.

Calculating How Many Calories
You Burn Per Day

Whether you're very lean, or have a lot of weight to lose, the Mifflin-St. Jeor Equation is considered the most accurate estimate of your resting metabolic rate (RMR), the number of calories you burn at rest[11-15].

Men's RMR = [4.5 x Pounds] + [16 x Inches] − [5 x Years] + 5

Women's RMR = [4.5 x Pounds] + [16 x Inches] − [5 x Years] − 161

If your BMI is over 35, these formulas may overestimate your RMR[16-17]. In this instance, simply multiply your RMR by 85% to get a more accurate estimate.

These formulas only let you know how many calories you burn just lying perfectly still for the entire day. To find the total number of calories you burn daily, you need your active metabolic rate (AMR), found by multiplying your RMR by one of the following factors based on your activity level:

1.2 to 1.3 = Couch potato with a desk job who sits most of the day

1.4 to 1.5 = Sitting half the day, and standing half the day

1.5 to 1.6 = Teacher, mechanic, salesperson, doctor, or nurse, standing most of the day

1.6 to 1.7 = Typical manual laborer who's moving around most of the day

1.8 to 1.9 = Very physically active job such as a dancer, farmer, or construction worker

1.9 to 2.0 = Extremely physically active work where you're on your feet and working hard all day

Let's calculate my AMR as an example. As of this writing, I weigh 160 pounds at 8% body fat. I'm thirty-two years old and five foot six inches tall (65.5 inches). My RMR is calculated as follows:

RMR = [4.5 x 160] + [16 x 66] − [5 x 32] + 5

= 720 + 1056 − 160 + 5 = 1,621 calories burned at rest over twenty-four hours.

Next, we find my AMR. I have a desk job and work out six hours a week. We're going to forget about my exercise, and just calculate my AMR factor as 1.25, a typical desk jockey's factor.

AMR = 1,641 x 1.25 = 2,051 calories burned per day

Obviously on the days I exercise, I'm burning more. We'll use this fact in one moment to figure out how to lose fat very easily. However, we won't be factoring excess post-exercise oxygen consumption (EPOC) into any of the caloric equations, even though that may raise my estimate by as much as 10%. Sometimes EPOC will boost your metabolism 5% for twelve hours, and other times 10% for twenty-four hours. This wild card will work in our favor whether we're factoring it in or not!

How to Cut Calories the Right Way

How do we cut calories the right way? The answer is simple. Your body only likes to increase or decrease calories in the short term, so only increase or decrease calories in the short term!

If you undereat by 10% to 20% fewer calories every day for four to six days, your body is *more* interested in stripping off body fat than stripping muscle. If you overeat by about 10% to 20% more calories every day for four to six days, your body is more interested in putting on lean tissue than laying on body fat. Therefore, to lose body fat while maintaining muscle and metabolism, undereat by 10% to 20% fewer calories for six days a week. Then for one day per week, overeat by the same amount to keep your metabolism from slowing.

To put it simply, you can only lose fat permanently by cutting calories temporarily.

Your overeating days are designed to fall on your carb-load days. You'll effectively be following the same routine for five or six days, and then carb loading with slightly higher calories for one to two days.

A more intuitive way to know when to carb load is to check your temperature every morning at the same time. It doesn't matter whether the average is 98 or 97.5, but whether that average varies by more than one degree. On the day when your temperature falls lower than 97 degrees, and it's usually above 97 degrees, it's time for a carb load.

For example, if you find that your temperature is a consistent 97.5 to 98 degrees for the last eight days, but your temperature drops to 96 on day nine, it's a sign that your metabolism has slowed. To get it back up, you'll want to increase your calories that day by 20%. Doing so will continue to push your metabolism up and up, so you don't have to cut so many calories to lose weight.

As a caveat to this principle, you will lose fat faster if you exercise to burn an extra 200 calories per day than if you were to simply cut 200 calories from your diet. The reason is that calories exercised away are much more likely to come from your fat stores than calories dieted away[25].

Let's Use Me Again to Calculate a Caloric Week's Worth of Fat Loss

You don't have to calculate how many calories per day you burn through exercise. Instead, eat at least 90% of the number of calories on your AMR, but *also* exercise four to seven days per week, for a total of five to ten hours of activity per week! That's it! The numbers will take care of themselves. In other words, if you eat a little less than your AMR *and* exercise, then you'll lose fat.

I'll prove to you that this works by actually calculating my total caloric burn for the days when exercising. A typical hour-long gym workout will burn around 0.15 times your RMR. Since I only work out for an hour, this adds an additional 230 calories on days that I exercise (0.15 x 2,050). That means I burn about 2,300 calories on exercise days, but only eat 2,050. I've cut my calories by a modest 8%.

If I had a lot of fat to lose, I could multiply my AMR by 90%, which is 1,850 calories, and eat that many calories per day while exercising the rest of the fat away. It doesn't have to be harder than that.

In short, if you want to lose fat, calculate your AMR, multiply it by 0.9, eat that many calories, but exercise four to seven days per week.

Why Is Weight Loss So Damn Hard?

Imagine that two years from now, you've gone from 250 pounds to 150 pounds. Your blood sugar is under control, and you're off all medications for diabetes. Congratulations! From a caloric perspective, how hard will it be for you to maintain a 100 pound weight loss? Unfortunately, not as easy as if you had always weighed 150 pounds. But knowing why can reveal exactly how to pull it off.

First and foremost, you'd need to continue following a low-carb diet cyclically, exercising, and taking your fish oil for the rest of your life. However, as a formerly overweight individual, your metabolism is not necessarily the same as someone's who never had to diet a day in their life. Several studies show that formerly obese individuals who have maintained a weight loss of more than 10% of their body weight must consume at least 15% fewer calories than those who never had to diet to maintain their weight[1], and will remain that way long term[4]. This was even true while they exercised. The reason is that formerly obese individuals waste far fewer calories as heat.

One study compared people who lost roughly 15% to 34% of their weight to obese individuals, and confirmed, as previously noted, that the now leaner individuals had slower metabolisms, burning on average 25% fewer calories than expected![3] They were simply expelling less energy over the day compared to what others of their same body weight and body fat would be spending. Just moving around, these formerly obese individuals burned fewer calories sitting, standing, or watching TV[5].

We call this moving around nonexercise activity thermogenesis (NEAT) to distinguish it from calories burned while exercising (I guess that would be called EAT). NEAT helps explain why lean individuals burn more calories than many obese individuals. They fidget more. After a large meal, they're more prone to talk more, stand up, play a game, or go for a walk. All those little activities add up to do some big caloric burn-offs. If you want to think about it in terms of math, the formerly obese and normal individual's RMRs and AMRs are the same, but the leaner individuals will voluntarily and subconsciously want to move more, resulting in more calories burned at the end of the day.

In one study, lean individuals were fed an extra 1,000 calories per day to try to fatten them up[6]. The ones who gained the least amount of weight were the ones who expelled the most calories via NEAT by standing, fidgeting, maintaining posture, etc. The researchers concluded "these results suggest that as humans overeat, activation of NEAT dissipates excess energy to preserve leanness, and that failure to activate NEAT may result in ready fat gain."

Basically, when overfed, lean individuals spend that energy faster and in greater amounts than overweight individuals who tend to move around less.

By the genetic luck of the draw, lean individuals waste far more calories every day than obese individuals. That slice of pizza you just ate? Your lean twin could waste 40% of those calories and never absorb it. He'll fidget more after eating it. He'll move around a little more than you. You, on the other hand, might efficiently store nearly every single calorie of that Italian delight as fat to survive the impending famine from the next ice age that your hypothalamus is expecting *any* minute. To use another analogy, those with less NEAT are like the lottery winners who put all their money in the bank, right into storage. They are saving for a rainy day. But the lean people with a lot of NEAT are the ones who go out and buy the yacht and Ferrari as soon as they win.

NEAT may in part be blamed on a genetic dopamine deficiency found in many overweight people. You might recall that dopamine is involved in motivation and reward. One study did find that the greater someone's BMI, the more deficient they were in a particular dopamine receptor[7]. Since dopamine is involved in energy output, it might also explain less NEAT in overweight individuals. It may also mean leaner people have a greater adrenal output, so they are utilizing more HSL after eating by fidgeting, moving around, or other subconscious movements.

> **Lack of dietary thermogenesis is truly one of a few genetic predispositions for obesity[2] – but not one that can't be beaten. To beat it is simple. If you're prone to moving less, then move more! Just keep exercising every day. 'Nuff said.**

So What's It Going to Really Take to Lose All That Weight and Keep It Off?

> **Now here is the good news. While there are many reasons you may not have a fast metabolism from birth, there are also many ways you can acquire a much faster one through knowledge and application.**

Research validates that losing weight and keeping it off is synonymous with reversing leptin resistance[21]. By cycling your carbs, and supplementing with fish oil and 5-HTP, you've got leptin covered.

Granted, formerly obese people may always waste fewer calories as heat after weight loss even when compared to controls with the same body fat percentage. However, a lot of these studies deal in weight loss instead of fat loss. There is a big difference. Weight loss entails losing fat, muscle, and water. Since muscle burns a lot of calories per day while fat burns next to none, losing muscle while losing fat is a guaranteed way to burn far fewer calories as the studies have shown. A 10% weight reduction was found to require roughly a decrease of 3.5 +/- 2.5 calories per pound of lean tissue to maintain[3]. Other studies have shown the more weight you have to lose, or the slower you try to lose it, the more fat as opposed to muscle you'll lose[8-10.] Typically, losing three or fewer pounds per week in the beginning, and one to two afterwards is not so fast that you'll lose muscle, but *only* if you lift weights!

So how do you lose the weight and keep it off? Simple!

1. Follow a low-carb diet because it reverses insulin resistance, and has been found to be more satiating than a low-fat diet.

2. Eat lots of protein because protein has a higher thermic effect of food than fat or carbohydrates (roughly 30% of calories wasted as heat compared to 10% for fat and carbs).

3. Perform high-intensity interval training to increase EPOC and lower insulin resistance by enhancing GLUT.

4. Avoid high-fructose corn syrup and highly glycemic or refined carbohydrates because they negatively influence leptin.

5. Drink green tea over coffee to increase dietary thermogenesis as much as 5%.

6. Eat frequent small meals with fiber, including glucomannan, and protein to further enhance satiety.

7. Supplement with fish oil to lower insulin resistance, increase dietary thermogenesis, and, extremely important, to increase leptin levels while on a low-carb diet.

8. Take three to six grams of CLA and 600 to 900 mg of GLA each day to blunt fat gain from inevitable overeating done from time to time.

9. Supplement with 5-HTP to increase leptin by raising insulin, and tyrosine as an insurance policy against overeating.

10. Lift weights to gain muscle, increasing your RMR and how many calories you burn per day. Train in a circuit fashion using whole-body exercises to use the most muscle at a time. Perform HIIT three or more times per week. The more activity you add in a day, the better.

Let's say you go from 250 pounds at 50% body fat to 150 pounds at 25% body fat. A worst-case scenario rule of thumb is that such a profound weight loss is costing you about six calories per pound of lean body weight to maintain your new weight compared to someone who has always weighed 150. With 112.5 pounds of lean tissue on your current frame, you're potentially burning 675 fewer calories per day than anyone your weight is expected to burn.

So let's do the math to see how we can offset this possible 675-calorie cost of admission to the land of lean. First, if you gained ten pounds of muscle, and lost ten more pounds of fat, you'd be 150 pounds at 18.3% body fat. That change alone could mitigate more than 150 calories per day of your loss.

Second, intense exercise done for fewer than twenty minutes three times per week can induce an EPOC that raises your metabolism a good 10% over forty-eight hours. If you burn as few as ten calories per pound of body weight, you would still be burning an extra 150 calories per day more by including this form of exercise, costing you one hour per week of your time.

Third, drinking green tea will earn you another 75. Further, adding fiber to every meal will knock off as much as 100 calories from the total amount you actually absorb. So far, we've hedged 475 calories from your daily loss. There are 200 to go.

Eating more protein and fewer carbs will increase the thermic effect of your food some. In fact, in one study, total calories wasted as heat were twice as high following a high-protein meal compared to one high in carbohydrates[18]. By eating 150 grams of protein per day for 600 calories, and conservatively assuming a 20% thermic effect instead of the standard 30%, you can safely waste 120 calories as heat. That leaves 80 calories. Park your car five minutes from your work, and take the stairs instead of the elevator, and you're done.

> **Any weight loss you make on this program is attainable and** *maintainable.*

The point of this exercise was not to calculate down to the kilocalorie every pound you could gain or lose. I didn't even include all the benefits of fish oil, 5-HTP, or tyrosine. The fish oil alone might take care of more than 75% of the potential caloric loss. The weight training and other exercise could very well bring your metabolism on par with someone naturally lean. Regardless, as a whole, the 10 strategies above will help you hold your ground as you lose weight, and keep you losing weight the longer you keep at it.

> **Living in this world of possibilities where long-term leanness is possible is the mindset you'll have to adopt to make it a reality. Know you can do this. Know it is possible. Then ask yourself how you can make it happen. This book is part of that answer. Follow the steps in this book every day. Then do it again the next. In a year from now, you'll wake up to a whole new you.**

The Eighth Prescription in Summary

- The quality of food matters just as much as the number of carbs and calories.
- You don't gain weight from how many calories you eat. Instead, you gain weight from how many of those calories you absorb.

- The average person wastes 10% of their fat calories, 10% of their carbohydrate calories, and a whopping 30% of their protein calories as heat.
- Eat five to six times a day, every two to three hours, making breakfast your largest meal.
- On your high-carb days, it is better for you to eat your highest-carb meals in the morning and go low carb at night because you are the most insulin sensitive in the morning.
- Your body only likes to increase or decrease calories in the short term, so only increase or decrease calories in the short term.
- Formerly obese individuals waste far fewer calories as heat, so they need to move more and eat better to make up for this metabolic disadvantage.

NINTH PRESCRIPTION

Know Your Diabetic Complications, Their Medications, and Your Alternatives

When It Comes to Using Prescription Medications, Don't Buy the Lie

To avoid some unnecessary controversy, let me start off by stating that I am not against prescription medication. I am for doing everything within our own power to treat ourselves without medication first. Only when that proves to be not enough or when faced with acute, life-threatening conditions should we take prescription meds. I have two reasons. First, many meds, especially those given to diabetics, treat the symptoms instead of the causes. Only a few drugs out there actually attempt to take a shot at reversing metabolic syndrome. Second, many drugs have side effects that can be as infuriating as the conditions they treat.

When weight loss can effectively "cure" diabetes, but most drugs for type II diabetes cause weight gain, I become infuriated. I don't believe there is any conspiracy at work—it is simply the nature of the drugs. If you increase insulin output, blood sugar will lower, but weight will rise. Meanwhile, if you increase insulin sensitivity, blood sugar will lower, and weight will lower. You get the same primary effect without the undesired secondary effect. That's why drugs like Metformin, Byetta, and Januvia are wonderful. They won't get in your way of trying to "cure" yourself naturally through weight loss.

However, if you take a class of drugs known as an insulin secretagogue, it's a different story. They will certainly lower blood sugar, but they make weight loss harder, making getting off the drug harder. Your doctor might tell you that your diabetes is so far advanced that it's either this powerful drug or insulin for you, and from their vantage point, they'd be right. They're neither expecting nor used to patients with advanced diabetes telling them that they want to do everything possible to stay off meds. Most patients don't even realize the full scope of their disease to understand why that decision is desirable or even possible. However, if you are such a patient who is willing to take the time and effort to make weight loss and a healthy lifestyle your primary mode of healing, I see no reason why your doctor should not give you the benefit of the doubt and help you by monitoring your blood work, lowering your meds as needed, and changing prescriptions to avoid complications like fatigue and weight gain.

However, there is a very important caveat to that decision. You *have* to follow through. You're literally playing with your life by turning down medication *if* you don't also make the changes in your lifestyle to heal. Take the meds, treat yourself without meds, do a combination of the two, but *do* something.

> **The cost of adopting a more natural approach is not cheap. It requires paying meticulous attention to what goes on inside, and how you treat your body. Are you willing to exercise? Are you willing to take supplements? Are you willing to indulge in certain foods and alcohol only occasionally? If so, then you will reap the payoffs with greater energy and nearly no side effects.**

When it comes to prescription drugs, the most insidious lie is that drugs are always necessary, and natural remedies do not work even a fraction as well. Continue to believe that, and the drug companies own you; your quality of life is forever doomed to remain far lower than you'd like.

The Drugs That Make You Fat

Many prescription medications can make fat loss harder for various reasons. The most common culprits are[1]:

- Nonsteroidal anti-inflammatory drugs (NSAIDs).
- Antihistamines.
- Estrogens and most synthetic hormone replacement therapies (HRTs), including birth control pills.
- Antidepressants.
- Insulin, insulin-stimulating drugs, and other diabetic drugs.
- Antiarthritis medications, steroids, and cortisone.
- Diuretics, beta-blockers, and other blood pressure medications.
- Sleeping pills and tranquilizers.

Estrogens, HRTs, and birth control pills are great examples of how medications affect fat loss. Estrogen causes fat gain by lowering thermogenesis. Fat gain increases estrogen, which in turn causes more fat. It's interesting to note that many farmers feed their cattle estrogen to fatten them up! Think about that; of all the drugs available to a farmer to fatten up cattle, estrogen is the one that works best. Tells you something, doesn't it?

Diabetics are often prescribed powerful combinations of oral and injectable medications that they are told they'll need to be on for the rest of their life. In the absence of a low-carb diet and exercise, I believe this would certainly be the case. However, consider the success that the late Dr. Robert Atkins had with many type II diabetics. In the *Atkins Diabetes Revolution*, the authors explain how he would treat diabetes with Metformin if needed and insulin when only absolutely necessary[4]. He was able to get several patients who were on insulin completely off it, no matter how advanced their diabetes. While he did not succeed 100% of the time, in many cases, he was able to significantly reduce if not altogether eliminate the need for diabetic, heart, and blood pressure medications.

Drugs Used to Treat Diabetes: The Good, the Bad, and the Ugly

Sulfonylureas (Insulin Secretagogues)[2-3] stimulate your pancreas to make more insulin. Among these are: Diabinese, Tolinase, Glucotrol, Orinase, Amaryl, Diabeta, Micronase, Glibenclamide, and Gliclazide. While they do lower blood sugar when taken initially, the side effects include weight gain, fluid retention, hypoglycemia, loss of effectiveness over time (meaning more drugs are needed), and they may increase the risk of a heart attack.

Meglitinides[2-3] (Non-Sulfonylurea Insulin Secretagogues) work like sulfonylureas to make your pancreas produce more insulin, though through a different mechanism. Among these are: Starlix, Prandin, and Mitiglinide. While they work faster than sulfonylureas, they have the very same side effects.

Biguanides[2-3] include only Metformin at the moment (Phenformin was removed from the market after it was believed to cause some deaths). It causes weight loss, generally does not cause hypoglycemia (but it sometimes did with me), and improves cholesterol, but it can be fatal in those with kidney disease and congestive heart failure (it does *not* cause these conditions).

Thiazolidinediones[2-3] (say it ten times fast!) increase insulin sensitivity. Among these are: Avandia and Actos, but Avandia may have already been pulled from the market by this publication due to its higher correlation with congestive heart failure, heart attack, and death compared to other diabetic drugs. Side effects include weight gain, fluid retention, anemia, liver problems, and potential heart problems.

Carbohydrate Absorption Blockers[2] do what their name says—they block the absorption of carbohydrates. Among those are: Precose and Glyset. These are safe, and cause neither hypoglycemia nor weight gain, but they may not lower the hA1c much and can cause upset stomach or gas (though I did not find this to be true when taking either).

Insulin[2-4] may be needed if your diabetes has progressed so far that your pancreas produces little or no insulin. A low-carb diet, exercise, and targeted supplementation may very well make the need for insulin unnecessary, but it is literally a life saver when and while needed. The greatest side effects are hypoglycemia and weight gain.

Incretin Enhancers[2-3] enhance the effect of incretins, gut hormones that rise in response to food, and work with insulin to lower blood sugar. Among these are: Januvia and Galvus (may not yet be FDA approved). They do not cause hypoglycemia or weight gain.

Incretin Hormone Mimetics[2] like Byetta mimic the incretin hormones instead of enhancing what is already indigenously available. It causes significant and sustained weight loss, reduced appetite, does not increase hypoglycemia, but may increase nausea when initiating therapy.

Blood Pressure Medications Known to Cause Weight Gain and Fatigue

Thiazides[2-3] are diuretics that can actually cause diabetes by increasing insulin resistance. Some of the better known are: Naturetin, Exna, Diurigen, Diuril, Hygroton, Thalitone, Esidrex, Ezide, Hydrodiuril, Hydro-Par, Microzide, Oretic, Diucardin, Saluron, Lozol, Aquatensen, Enduron, Mykrox, Zaroxolyn, Renese, Hydromox, Diurese, Metahydrin, and Naqua.

Beta-Blockers[2-4] block the beta receptors in your heart to relax blood vessels and slow heart rate. However, beta receptors are also on fat cells and responsible for fat release. Block a beta receptor and you block fat loss. Tenormin (I personally know someone who gained thirty pounds after losing fifty on a low-carb diet once they started this drug), Normodyne, Trandate, Lopressor, Toprol, Corgard, Levatol, Inderal, Betapace, Sorine, and Blocadren are some of the better known beta-blockers.

Don't Take a Drug You Don't Have to Take

Talk to your doctor about your concerns with weight gain and other unwanted side effects. Ask about natural over synthetic forms, lower dosages, and other forms of the medication like a patch, pill, or injection. However, be sure your doctor is first open to natural "cures", and second, familiar with them. I am amazed how one doctor thinks all natural "cures" are bogus, while another embraces them. After all, they both went to med school...

Work with your doctor to slowly reduce the dosage until the drug is no longer needed. The idea is to get your diet, exercise, and stress all under control while religiously taking supplements that have been proven to make a difference in your condition, *ensuring that it does not worsen.* Your doctor wants this above all else, and careful and frequent monitoring may be needed to make this happen. While you may never totally get off the medication, you may be able to lower the dosage to the point that you notice zero side effects, including weight gain.

A good diet, regular exercise, enough sleep, and less stress have a tremendous impact on the severity of many conditions like diabetes, hypertension, arthritis, high cholesterol, and heart disease to name a few. Yes, all that stuff you've been reading about really does make a difference in your health! Lifestyle, which includes everything but the Rx, can do a few things for your med dosage, from making them completely unnecessary to requiring a far lower dosage.

Get your lifestyle under control.

Supplements That Can Reduce the Need for Medications

Below are several groups of supplements that have a synergistic effect on one or more aspects of diabetes. Since there are literally thousands of supplements discovered so far that can improve diabetes, this list is neither an exhaustive nor complete picture of everything you could be taking that might work. Instead, my aim was to give you a list of the most effective and most studied supplements available without prescription, that you could use to wean yourself off blood sugar, cholesterol, blood pressure, and heart medication, *or at the very least reduce your dosages.* As a plus, most of them help with weight loss as well.

However, if you are already on such medications, you're absolutely going to need the help of a complementary physician familiar with these supplements and others to delicately and systematically lower your medications. They'll also need to check the below recommendations for contraindications against certain drugs you're taking.

For example, fish oil can thin the blood, so you'd need to tell your doctor you're taking it if you're on blood thinners. Some recommendations below might not be appropriate if you're pregnant or nursing. The combination of vanadium and an insulin secretagogue could give your blood sugar a wallop, lowering it too much too fast. This is why adding a little vanadium, and lowering a little medication is the right way to go. Your doctor should be familiar with supplements, use them in their practice, and be willing to help wean you off medications where possible.

If you already have high blood pressure, you'll need to consult with a physician prior to using tyrosine or phenylalanine, as both these amino acids can increase it. If they say to stay away, for enhanced energy and fat burning, use yerba maté tea instead, a member of the methylxanthine family that causes smooth muscle relaxation (lowers blood pressure)[47] Green tea works for the same reason.

Be prepared for your doctor's opinion. Most important, should yours think all supplements are garbage, you have two choices: you can ask her why she thinks that, or you can find another one with a different opinion. This may all seem like too much of a hassle, but it will be well worth it when you're lighter and on little or no medication.

> **For a list of doctors with a focus on nutrition, visit the American College for Advancement in Medicine at http://www.acam.org or the American Society of Bariatric Physicians at http://www.asbp.org.**

Please remember the goal of these supplements is meant to assist your efforts with cutting carbs and exercising, not replace them. To fix your weight-loss woes from medications, the combination of diet and exercise must be strong enough to reduce your need for these meds. Low-carb diets reduce the prescription need for diabetes, heart disease, high cholesterol, and high blood pressure. Using far less alcohol and illicit drugs and quitting smoking will also go a long way. There is no magic pill, formed neither by nature nor a pharmaceutical company, that can "cure" diabetes by itself. Fish oil is the closest, but more is needed than even that. Always remember, if you think you can do this for the rest of your life, it's possible.

Take these supplements a little at a time. Have a few with your first and fourth meals, second and fifth meals, and third and sixth meals.

Multivitamin, Vitamin D, & Probiotics: You need a quality multivitamin to cover any deficiencies that you may have. There is a lot of new research that shows vitamin D may help with your blood sugar and blood pressure. Even if you work outside in the sun, you may still be deficient. To learn more, visit http://www.VitaminDCouncil.org.

Probiotics contain beneficial bacteria including acidophilus that can keep your entire GI tract healthy, not to mention prevent and fight any yeast problems that may be developing there. Since fungal infections feed on sugar, and can lead to sugar cravings, ensuring you're preventing a treatable and unnecessary reason for emotionally eating is vital. Take the multivitamin as directed, and add 4,000 IU of vitamin D plus 4 billion cells of beneficial bacteria each day.

Chromium and Vanadium[5-12]**:** Both reduce blood sugar and improve insulin sensitivity. They've also been proven important for treating hypertension and high cholesterol. Take 400 mcg of chromium and 20 mcg of vanadium twice per day with food.

Pantethine[13-17]: A potent cholesterol-fighting agent. It raises HDL, and lowers LDL and VLDL (triglycerides). Take 300 mg three times per day.

Alpha Lipoic Acid[18-21]**:** Extremely effective at lowering insulin resistance. It also lessens nerve pain, but does not repair nerve damage, and can take up to three months to work. Get 300 mg twice per day with meals for nerve pain, and up to 1,000 mg per day for blood sugar control.

L-Taurine[22-25]**:** A natural diuretic that lowers blood pressure and improves insulin sensitivity. Get 1,000 mg three times per day on an empty stomach.

Magnesium, Calcium, & Vitamin B$_6$[26-32]**:** Strengthens the heart, lowers blood pressure, and is often deficient in diabetics. It's also effective at improving insulin sensitivity, especially when taken with vanadyl sulfate. Calcium helps make insulin and should be taken to balance out magnesium. Vitamin B$_6$ is a synergist of magnesium and is also helpful for eye health. Get 1,000 mg of magnesium, 500 mg of calcium, and 200 mg of B_6 at night with food.

CoQ10[33-40] and L-carnitine[41-43]: These two are the heart patient's best friends. Coenzyme Q-10 (CoQ10) helps people with congestive heart failure, cardiomyopathies, or angina, all by increasing the heart's ability to function with reduced oxygen, pumping more blood to major organs, and increasing energy production in cardiac cells. It also lowers blood sugar. However, it unfortunately drops with age, making CoQ10 all the more important to add as a supplement. L-carnitine protects the heart, lowers cholesterol, boosts energy, and burns fat, especially when combined with CoQ10. Get 2,000 mg of L-carnitine and 100 mg of CoQ10 twice per day with meals.

Inositol, Biotin and Vitamin C[44]: A must for diabetic neuropathy - they ease nerve pain and improve nerve function. Vitamin C is a master antioxidant involved with virtually every metabolic function, and helps you avoid losing inositol in the first place. They speed fat loss by increasing fat-burning enzymes, and biotin also helps reverse insulin resistance. Get 15 mg of biotin, 1,500 mg of inositol, and 2,000 mg of vitamin C per day.

Omega-3s[45] with Vitamin E and Selenium: The laundry list of benefits from taking fish oil and flaxseeds seems endless.

- Improved insulin sensitivity and more stable blood sugar.
- Faster metabolism, greater fat loss, and less hunger.
- Lower blood pressure and improved cholesterol.
- Improved kidney function.
- Less nerve pain from neuropathy.
- Increased energy and concentration.
- Fewer bouts and less severity of depression due to increased serotonin levels.
- Higher testosterone and growth hormone levels, a good thing for women as well.
- Fewer PMS symptoms, a good thing for men as well.

- Less inflammation, preventing disease and promoting healing.
- *And the list goes on…*

Vitamin E and selenium are key antioxidants that reduce inflammation to improve blood sugar and lipid profiles. Vitamin E should be taken any time you're using fish oil in your diet because fish oil is unstable and may degrade in the bottle. Vitamin E safeguards you against this potential threat while selenium makes the vitamin E more effective. For the same reason, store all fish oils in your fridge once opened. Get at least 4,000 mg of a combination of EPA and DHA, plus four tablespoons of flaxseeds daily. In addition, take 400 IU of vitamin E with 100 mcg of Selenium twice per day with food.

CLA and GLA**:** Helps the body turn excess calories into muscle instead of fat, and prevents regaining weight after dieting. Take two grams of CLA twice per day and 300 mg of GLA two to three times per day with food.

Four great resources that list most of the proven natural remedies for nearly any disease are:
- *The Encyclopedia of Natural Medicine* by Michael Murray, N.D., and Joseph Pizzorno, N.D.
- *The Dr. Atkins' Vita-Nutrient Solution* by Dr. Robert Atkins.
- *Prescription for Nutritional Healing* by Phyllis and James Balch.
- Visit http://www.nutros.com for a complete explanation on most supplements and which conditions they treat.

You Don't Need a Fat Wallet to Lose Fat

If you find your pocketbook running thin, buy fish oil and a good multivitamin with antioxidants first. Glucomannan and flaxseeds are very cheap, as are CLA and GLA. Shop around online for bargains. I recommend http://www.vitacost.com. If you'd like to find natural sources of most of the nutrients below, visit http://www.nutritiondata.com. More information on each supplement can be found online at http://www.nutros.com. Consult with your accountant and start an HSA (health savings account) so that you can purchase all your supplements and medications with before-tax dollars.

Other Helpful Fats and Fibers

Organic Virgin Coconut Oil[46]**:** The very best oil to cook with! It contains the healthy saturated fat lauric acid, rich in medium chain triglycerides (MCTs). Unlike normal fats, MCTs are immediately burned by the liver for energy, making them far less likely to be stored as fat. MCTs also increase energy, and may even increase resting metabolic rate. Because coconut oil is over 50% MCTs, and you'll be using it while on a low-carb diet, its saturated fat will not contribute to cholesterol, and in fact will raise good HDL cholesterol. Use it instead of butter in any recipe (never use margarine no matter what).

Olive Oil: Another great oil for the heart that also fights cholesterol. Get one tablespoon per day with meals.

Glucomannan: The most insoluble of insoluble fibers! Use this fiber powder in smoothies, soup, chili, sauces, eggs, and anything else you can think of. The result will be more fullness and fewer calories! Shoot for ten to fifteen grams for men and eight to twelve grams for women per day.

Psyllium Husks: Soluble and insoluble fiber that lowers cholesterol, improves satiety, relieves constipation, and lowers blood sugar. Use only if unable to achieve twenty-five to thirty-five grams of fiber per day from vegetables, flaxseeds, and glucomannan. Mix one tablespoon with sixteen ounces of water. Don't take your supplements or oral medications within two hours of having psyllium husks. The fiber may block the absorption of some of the nutrients. Fiber from food is a different story, and is OK to consume with oral medications and supplements.

Other Helpful Amino Acids and Herbs

L-Glutamine: Boosts energy and reduces carb cravings. Take 2,000 mg whenever cravings arise with or without food.

5-HTP: Reduces carb cravings. Take 25 to 400 mg as needed on an empty stomach. Consult a physician if considering more than 200 mg at a time. 100 mg can be taken with melatonin at bedtime for a more restful sleep.

L-Tyrosine and L-Phenylalanine: Reduces stress to lower blood sugar, gives energy, supports thyroid health, and suppresses appetite. Have 1,000 mg of each three times per day on an empty stomach.

L-Theanine: A natural antianxiety supplement that's naturally found in green tea and is responsible for the tea's energetic yet nonjittery effect. Take 100 mg when stressed. 100 mg can be taken with melatonin and 5-HTP at bedtime for a more restful sleep.

Melatonin: Best used at night for a restful night sleep. It's also vital if you suffer from nighttime eating syndrome. Try 0.5 mg per day and keep that dosage if you notice it solves your insomnia. Go as high as 3 mg per day if needed.

Two Drinks That Can Change Your Life: The NDP Shake and the Stress Buster

The easiest way to get your fish oil and 5-HTP while simultaneously controlling appetite and stress is in a formula I call the New Diabetes Prescription Shake. It is a convenient and good-tasting way to get your nutritional needs met, and it has a profound effect on your appetite, stress, and energy level.

The New Diabetes Prescription Super Shake

This recipe makes two shakes. Have one in the morning, and the other shake four or more hours later. Blend for one minute, let sit for three so the glucomannan can expand in water, and then blend for a minute more:

2-4 cups of water

2 scoops low-carb protein powder
  (vanilla flavor recommended)

4 teaspoons of Carlson Lab's The Very Finest Fish Oil

4 tablespoons of milled flaxseeds

½ tablespoon of glucomannan powder

200 mg of 5-HTP (100 mg if you get tired)

1 teaspoon of cinnamon

1 tablespoon nonalcohol vanilla bean extract

Stevia to taste

In addition to the shake, you should take 2,000 mg of CLA and 600 mg GLA (from borage oil).

Nutritional information per serving using two scoops Nature's Best Perfect Zero Carb Isopure Creamy Vanilla: 26 grams of protein, 14 grams of fat, 2 grams of carbohydrate, 6 grams of fiber, and 240 calories. Since the protein powder I use has zero carbs, be sure to add the carbs from the brand you use.

There are many flavors available, and many more possible combinations than you'll read about below. Truly, the only rule to coming up with your own version is to not add more than five carbs or fifty calories per shake compared to the plain version.

- **Strawberry**: Add 100 grams of strawberries (about six medium large berries). Adds three carbs, one gram of fiber, and twelve calories per shake.
- **Chocolate**: Add three tablespoons of organic cocoa powder. That should be the only ingredient on the can. How clear can I make it that this should not be chocolate syrup? Adds 1.5 grams of fat, 3.5 grams of protein, 2.5 grams of carbs, 4.5 grams of fiber, and 40 calories per shake.
- **Mocha**: Add three tablespoons of organic cocoa powder, but use decaffeinated coffee instead of water in the recipe. Adds 1.5 grams of fat, 3.5 grams of protein, 2.5 grams of carbs, 4.5 grams of fiber, and 40 calories per

shake.

- **Pumpkin**: Add ½ cup of raw canned pumpkin and pumpkin spice to taste. Adds 2 grams of carbs, 2 grams of fiber, and 10 calories.

Mix the ingredients together in a blender. More glucomannan and less water gives you a thick yogurt consistency when left to set overnight. For protein powder, I highly recommend Low Carb Metabolic Drive from https://www.t-nation.com/online-StoreSimple.jsp, Isopure Zero Carb Protein, or Designer Whey, both found at http://www.vitacost.com and most health food stores. When buying 5-HTP, get the kind where you can open the pill and pour the powder straight into the mixture. You can also add any supplements that you can break open and pour into the mixture except amino acids—they would be absorbed as food, lessening the desired effect.

The Stress-Buster Tonic

The easiest way to get your stress-controlling amino acids is to make the Stress Buster:

- 16-24 ounces of water.
- 4,000 - 6,000 mg of L-tyrosine.
- 4,000 - 6,000 mg of L-phenylalanine.
- 4,000 - 6,000 mg of L-glutamine.
- 100 - 200 mg of L-theanine.

The L-phenylalanine is optional, but strongly recommended if you're trying to quit drinking caffeinated coffee or smoking cigarettes. The Stress Buster should make you feel energized. If you at all feel sleepy, try using less of the L-theanine.

You can drink this in three ways. The first is plain, which is fine if you don't mind tasting the slight sweetness from the amino acids. You may taste nothing at all. The second way is by adding lemon juice and Stevia to taste. However, do not use Crystal Light or any other chemically laden drink that contains sugar, sugar alcohols, artificial sweeteners like Splenda, Sweet'n

Low, or Equal, or natural sweeteners like honey. Use Stevia or nothing at all. The third way is to make an ice tea from green tea and/or yerba maté tea, and pour the amino acids in there. Feel free to add the lemon juice or Stevia as well.

In either case, the Stress Buster works best without coffee or black tea of any kind. I highly recommend using it with the aforementioned green teas above. Try it for one week or even one day, and you'll notice a profound difference.

The Stress Buster is meant to be taken in two or three dosages. Don't drink it all at once! While getting that much of each amino acid will likely do no harm more than 99.99% of the time, by drinking it all at once you'll be wasting the effects of appetite control, energy, stress relief, and an overall sense of well-being that comes from using the Stress Buster at the worst times of the day —midafternoon and midmorning. Take one-third to one-half of the drink at those two times and see the difference. If you only take one-third at each of those times, late afternoon is another stressful time when the Stress Buster can work wonders. You'll get through each time much easier with far fewer cravings. It really is worth it.

Medications Should Not Interfere With Diabetes' Ultimate "Cure": Weight Loss

When the reasons for weight gain are not obvious, diabetic complications and their medications bear consideration. Sometimes the medications do more harm than good, and many times, you can kill the complications by changing prescriptions. The main side effect from changing is usually weight loss.

Consider my friend Jessica who lost sixty pounds in twelve months on a low-carb diet, only to regain fifteen pounds in fat and water after one month on a beta-blocker, Atenolol. If you have high blood pressure, a beta-blocker will certainly help you control that condition, but at the cost of weight gain and fatigue. What if, instead, you exercised five days a week, ate better, and consumed the amino acid L-taurine, a natural diuretic? This solution's direct effect on your blood pressure, plus its indirect effect via weight loss, is going to control your blood pressure better in the long run, and without the weight gain, fatigue, or copay. You decide how to treat your medications. Doctors don't decide—they prescribe. Learn your alternatives to drug therapy, and as a rule, choose it as a last result, and always alongside diet, exercise, natural supplements, and lifestyle.

One More Shameless Plug to Wear You Down

So if you were only going to buy one supplement, what would it be? I'll give you three hints… It swims… You eat it… The rich eat its unborn children… If you guessed fish oil, give yourself a gold star. If you didn't, reread the chapter.

The Ninth Prescription in Summary

- Drugs are not always necessary to heal from diabetes. Some of them make losing weight much harder.
- The most common kinds of drugs that cause fat gain and slow metabolism include nonsteroidal anti-inflammatory drugs (NSAIDs); antihistamines; estrogens and most synthetic hormone replacement therapies (HRTs), including birth control pills; antidepressants; insulin, insulin-stimulating drugs, and other diabetic drugs; antiarthritis medications, steroids, and cortisone; diuretics, beta-blockers, and other blood pressure medications; sleeping pills and tranquilizers.
- Above all else, you must work with your doctor and take controlling your diabetes with less or no medication extremely seriously. The ultimate goal far and away is to get blood sugar and all other diabetic complications under control.
- For a list of doctors with a focus on nutrition, visit the

American College for Advancement in Medicine at http://www.acam.org or the American Society of Bariatric Physicians at http://www.asbp.org.

- Check out the Twelfth Prescription for an hour-by-hour breakdown of what supplements to take and when.

TENTH PRESCRIPTION

Find Healthy Recipes That Taste Better Than Your Unhealthy Favorites

Recipes Even a Single Diabetic Parent of Four Could Prepare and Enjoy!

Most weekday low-carb recipes are made with the busy nine to five professional in mind. We all have commitments to our work, families, and now thanks to diabetes, our health. While there are tons of low-carb cookbooks available on the market, all full of delicious recipes, what can you cook for five or six meals when scraping even twenty minutes together to prepare seems like a major sacrifice? Pot roasts and salmon steaks, though undeniably delicious, take time. The easiest way to incorporate them into a busy workweek is to cook them on Sunday, and eat a serving each day. For that reason, you need recipes that can still taste great five days after cooking them!

Also, should a recipe's calorie or carbohydrate content be too high or too low for you, changing portion sizes to match your caloric needs, or removing some of the higher-carb ingredients, will in no way harm the positive effect that these recipes can have on your diabetes. Here's to your health!

Higher-Carb Recipes

Roasted Vegetables – *34 Carbs and 190 Calories*

6 red potatoes chopped into bite-sized pieces

1 chopped small red onion

1 sliced Anaheim chili pepper

1 chopped sweet red pepper

1 chopped yellow crookneck squash

$^1/_2$ chopped eggplant

2 ounces shredded Manchego cheese

Dash real salt

Dash cayenne pepper

Dash oregano

Olive oil cooking spray

Spray a skillet with olive oil and bring to medium heat. Sauté potatoes for 5 minutes, and then add onions, eggplant, peppers, squash, and seasonings. Once they begin to brown, mix in cheese until melted. Makes 6 servings. Nutritional information: 3 grams of fat, 7 grams of protein, 34 grams of carbohydrates, 6 grams of fiber, and 190 calories.

Crepes – *5 Carbs and 100 Calories*

Toppings

2 cups sliced strawberries

1 cup nonfat Greek Yogurt

Crepes

2 tablespoons melted butter

2 large eggs

4 tablespoons whole wheat flour

2 tablespoons extra-virgin olive oil

¼ cup half-and-half

½ cup water as needed

½ teaspoon Stevia

½ teaspoon salt

Whisk flour and eggs together in a large bowl. Gradually stir in water, butter, Stevia, and salt until smooth. Bring a skillet to medium heat and coat with olive oil. Pour ¼ cup of batter at a time into pan, tilting pan in circular motion to allow for faster, more even cooking. Heat for 2 minutes until bottom is a light golden brown. Loosen with spatula, turn over, and cook the other side. Set aside and add another ¼ cup of mixture until all crepes have been cooked. Coat the inside of each crepe with yogurt and berries. Makes 8 servings. Nutritional information: 7 grams of fat, 5 grams of protein, 5 grams of carbohydrates, 1 gram of fiber, and 100 calories.

Ezekiel Grilled Cheese Sandwich – *22 Carbs & 275 Calories*

2 slices of Ezekiel 4:9 bread

2 slices of low-fat Havarti cheese

Coat a skillet set on medium heat with olive oil cooking spray. Grill sandwich for 3 to 5 minutes until bottom is a light golden-brown. Flip and repeat. Makes 1 serving. Nutritional information: 11 grams of fat, 22 grams of protein, 22 grams of carbs, 6 grams of fiber, and 275 calories.

Omega Berry Oatmeal – *31 Carbs & 380 Calories*

½ cup steel cut Irish oatmeal

1 scoop low-carb whey or casein protein power

2 teaspoons of Carlson Lab's The Very Finest Fish Oil

2 tablespoons of milled flaxseeds

½ cup sliced strawberries

Stevia to taste

1 to 2 cups boiling water to desired thickness

Combine all ingredients save berries, and pour water to desired thickness. Stir for 60 seconds to allow thickening. Add berries and serve. Makes 1 serving. Nutritional information: 16 grams of fat, 28 grams of protein, 31 grams of carbohydrates, 7 grams of fiber, and 380 calories.

Almond Butter Apples – *20 Carbs & 300 Calories*

3 tablespoons of almond butter

1 large apple cut into slices

Dip apples into almond butter and enjoy. Makes 1 serving. Nutritional information: 20 grams of fat, 10 grams of protein, 20 grams of carbohydrates, 5 grams of fiber, and 300 calories.

Greek Yogurt & Cantaloupe – *29 Carbs & 240 Calories*

1 cup nonfat Greek yogurt

1 teaspoon honey

¼ teaspoon Stevia

1 teaspoon of Carlson Lab's The Very Finest Fish Oil

¼ chopped cantaloupe

Mix yogurt, honey, Stevia, and fish oil together. Place cantaloupe into mixture or dip in mixture. Makes 1 serving. Nutritional information: 4 grams of fat, 22 grams of protein, 29 grams of carbs, 2 grams of fiber, and 240 calories.

Happy Diabetic Cocoa – *8 Carbs & 100 Calories*

3 tablespoons organic raw cocoa

½ teaspoon Stevia

1 tablespoon alcohol-free vanilla extract

1 tablespoon heavy cream

Boiling water

Mix ingredients together, add water, and enjoy. Makes 1 serving. Nutritional information: 9 grams of fat, 5 grams of protein, 8 grams of carbohydrates, 9 grams of fiber, and 100 calories.

High-Protein Mocha Cappuccino – *12 Carbs & 280 Calories*

8 ounces hot decaf coffee (or half caffeinated and half decaf)

1 scoop chocolate or vanilla protein powder (Low Carb Metabolic Drive is recommended)

2 tablespoons heavy cream

3 tablespoons organic raw cocoa

1 tablespoon alcohol-free vanilla extract

Stevia to taste

½ teaspoon of glucomannan powder

Combine all ingredients and blend on medium for 4 minutes until smooth. Omit glucomannan for a thinner consistency. Makes 1 serving. Nutritional information: 15 grams of fat, 25 grams of protein, 12 grams of carbohydrates, 11 grams of fiber, and 280 calories.

Flat Bread Pesto Pizza – *18 Carbs & 480 Calories*

3 Mission Low Carb Balance Whole Wheat Tortillas (Large Burrito Size)

4 tablespoons of pesto

1 cup of shredded low-fat Italian cheeses

Coat a skillet with olive oil spray and set on medium heat. Spread 1 tortilla with pesto and cover with cheese. Place another tortilla on top, and again cover with pesto and then cheese. Cover with the third tortilla. Let cook for 3 to 5 minutes until bottom tortilla becomes golden and cheese begins to melt. Flip and cook for another 2 to 4 minutes. Cut into 8 pieces and enjoy. Makes 2 servings. Nutritional information: 30 grams of fat, 34 grams of protein, 18 grams of carbohydrates, 32 grams of fiber, and 480 calories.

Eggs, Toast, and Fruit – *40 Carbs & 485 Calories*

2 large eggs

2 slices of Ezekiel 4:9 bread

1 cup of sliced strawberries

1 tablespoon melted coconut butter

2 teaspoons of honey

Cook eggs any style desired, toast bread, and spread with coconut butter and honey. Makes 1 serving. Nutritional information:
25 grams of fat, 20 grams of protein, 40 grams of carbohydrates, 8
grams of fiber, and 485 calories.

Hummus, Veggies, Fruit, and Edamame – *23 Carbs & 240 Calories*

½ cup shelled edamame (baby soybeans)

¼ cup hummus dip

½ cup baby carrots

½ cup any melon

Dip carrots in hummus and enjoy. Makes 1 serving. Nutritional
information: 11 grams of fat, 13 grams of protein, 23 grams of carbohydrates, 9 grams of fiber, and 240 calories.

Turkey and Bean Chili – *25 Carbs & 295 Calories*

3 ounces lean ground turkey

¼ cup thawed green peas

½ cup rinsed and drained kidney beans

½ cup Bella Vita Low Carb Pasta Sauce, Tomato Basil
Style

½ teaspoon glucomannan powder

Coat a skillet with olive oil spray and set on medium heat. First,
cook turkey for 8 to 12 minutes until browned. Set aside, respray
skillet, and add peas, beans, and tomato sauce. Stir for 1 minute, and
then slowly stir in glucomannan powder for 1 more minute. Combine with turkey, let cool for 5 minutes, and serve. Makes one serving. Nutritional information: 6 grams of fat, 35 grams of protein, 25
grams of carbohydrates, 14 grams of fiber, and 295 calories.

Bison Chili – *5 Carbs & 140 Calories*

1½ pounds ground bison

2 tablespoons extra-virgin coconut oil

1 diced onion

½ cup chopped red and green peppers

3 minced cloves of garlic

1 pound pinto beans

1½ pound chopped tomatoes

Sea salt

Black pepper

2 tablespoons chili powder

½ teaspoon oregano powder

2 teaspoons cumin

2 tablespoons lemon juice

1 tablespoon glucomannan powder

Heat the bison in 1 tablespoon of coconut oil in a skillet set on medium heat. Season with salt and pepper. Cook for 5 minutes, stirring the whole time until bison is light brown. Set aside. In a large pot set on medium heat, add remaining coconut oil plus onions, peppers, and garlic. Cook for 4 to 6 minutes before adding beans, tomatoes, chili powder, oregano, and cumin. Reduce heat to low, cover, and cook for half an hour. Now add bison and lemon juice. Slowly stir in glucomannan using a whisk to avoid clumping. Leave uncovered, and cook for 15 more minutes, occasionally stirring to let glucomannan continue expanding and thickening the sauce. Makes 6 servings. Nutritional information: 10 grams of fat, 7 grams of protein, 5 grams of carbohydrate, 3 grams of fiber, and 140 calories.

Sandwich and Salad Recipes

Omega-3 Caesar Dressing – *1.5 Carbs & 180 Calories*

¼ cup mayonnaise

2 teaspoons lemon juice

1 teaspoon Worcestershire sauce

2 pressed garlic cloves

2 tablespoons Carlson Lab's The Very Finest Fish Oil

2 tablespoons Parmesan cheese

Using a food processor, process mayo, lemon juice, Worcestershire sauce, and garlic cloves first before adding fish oil and cheese. Blend until smooth. Makes 4 servings, netting about 2,000 mg of EPA and DHA. Nutritional information (2 tablespoons): 18 grams of fat, 1 gram of protein, 1.5 grams of carbohydrates, 0 fiber, and 180 calories.

Omega-3 Lemon Vinaigrette Dressing – *1 Carb & 175 Calories*

⅛ cup wine vinegar

1 teaspoon Dijon mustard

¼ teaspoon salt

⅛ teaspoon pepper

1 teaspoon grated lemon rind

1 tablespoon finely chopped shallot

⅛ cup Carlson Lab's The Very Finest Fish Oil

¼ cup extra-virgin olive oil

Whisk all ingredients together in a container that can be covered and refrigerated (or store in a bottle in fridge). Makes 4 servings, netting 2,000 mg of EPA and DHA per serving. Nutritional information (2 tablespoons): 19 grams of fat, 0 grams of protein, 1 gram of carbohydrate, 0 grams of fiber, and 175 calories.

Omega-3 Italian Dressing – *1 Carb & 140 Calories*

1 tablespoon white wine vinegar

¼ cup Carlson Lab's The Very Finest Fish Oil

¼ cup heavy cream

¼ cup olive oil mayonnaise

¼ teaspoon salt

¼ teaspoon pepper

1 garlic clove

1 teaspoon Italian seasoning

Whisk all ingredients together in a container that can be covered and refrigerated (or store in a bottle in fridge). Makes 8 servings, netting 2,000 mg of EPA and DHA per serving. Nutritional information (2 tablespoons): 14 grams of fat, 0 grams of protein, 1 gram of carbohydrate, 0 grams of fiber, and 140 calories.

Chef Salad with Omega-3 Italian Dressing – *3 Carbs & 310 Calories*

2 ounces chopped nitrate-free deli ham (only ingredients should be ham and salt)

¼ cup low-fat mixed cheese

1 ounce low-fat Swiss cheese

2 ounces chopped cucumber

2 ounces chopped romaine lettuce

2 ounces Omega-3 Italian Dressing

Add ingredients together in bowl, toss, and serve. Makes 1 serving. Nutritional information: 22 grams of fat, 24 grams of protein, 3 grams of carbohydrates, 1 gram of fiber, and 310 calories.

Spinach Salad with Omega-3 Lemon Vinaigrette Dressing – *3 Carbs & 350 Calories*

2 ounces of organic spinach

3 ounces grilled chopped chicken breast

1 ounce crumbled feta cheese

2 ounces Omega-3 Lemon Vinaigrette Dressing

Add ingredients together in bowl, toss, and serve. Makes 1 serving. Nutritional information: 24 grams of fat, 30 grams of protein, 3 grams of carbohydrates, 5 grams of fiber, and 350 calories.

Chicken Caesar Salad with Omega-3 Caesar Dressing – *3 Carbs & 310 Calories*

2 ounces of Caesar salad leaves

3 ounces of grilled chicken breast cut into strips

2 tablespoons Parmesan cheese

2 ounces Omega-3 Caesar Dressing

Add ingredients together in bowl, toss, and serve. Makes 1 serving. Nutritional information: 23 grams of fat, 25 grams of protein, 3 grams of carbohydrates, 2 grams of fiber, and 310 calories.

Low-Carb Macadamia Nut Butter and Honey Sandwich – 10 Carbs & 270 Calories

2 slices low-carb bread (after subtracting fiber from total carb count, there should only be 1 or 2 "net" carbs left over – fiber does not count as a carbohydrate)

2 tablespoons organic natural macadamia butter (macadamias and water should be only ingredients)

2 teaspoons organic raw honey (be careful measuring out the honey; it is extremely dense and easy to use too much).

On each slice of bread, smear first the nut butter, and then the honey over it. Press together and enjoy. Nutritional information (using Julian Bakery's* low carb flax bread): 22 grams of fat, 7 grams of protein, 10 grams of carbohydrates, 17 grams of fiber, and 270 calories.

* to order from Julian Bakery online, visit http://www.julianbakery.com

Low-Carb Grilled Cheese Sandwich – 3 Carbs & 270 Calories

2 slices low-carb bread (after subtracting fiber from total carb count, there should only be 1 or 2 "net" carbs left over – fiber does not count as a carbohydrate)

2 slices low-fat Swiss, or cheddar cheese

2 tablespoons coconut oil

Melt one tablespoon of coconut oil in skillet. Once melted, place cheese between bread and place in skillet. Press down with spatula a few times, and once bread is golden brown, melt second tablespoon of coconut oil, flip sandwich, and heat other side until golden brown. Let cool for 5 minutes and serve. Nutritional information (using Julian Bakery's low-carb flax bread): 20 grams of fat, 20 grams of protein, 3 grams of carbohydrates, 15 grams of fiber, and 270 calories.

Low-Carb Ham and Cheese Sandwich –
3 Carbs & 200 Calories

   2 slices low-carb bread (after subtracting fiber from total
      carb count, there should only be 1 or 2 "net" carbs left
      over – fiber does not count as a carbohydrate)

   2 slices low-fat Swiss, cheddar, or other cheese

   2 ounces nitrate-free deli ham

   Lettuce, mustard, and other carb-free garnishes as desired
      (be wary of mayonnaise – it will add calories)

   Place ham, cheese, and other ingredients between bread and
enjoy. Nutritional information (using Julian Bakery's low-carb flax
bread): 10 grams of fat, 25 grams of protein, 3 grams of carbohydrates, 15 grams of fiber, and 200 calories.

Meat and Fish Recipes

Grilled Salmon with Garlic Spinach –
2 Carbs & 300 Calories

   1 pound fresh Atlantic salmon

   1 pounds fresh spinach

   2 pressed cloves of garlic

   1 tablespoon Italian seasoning

   ¼ teaspoon Stevia

   ½ teaspoon salt

   ⅛ teaspoon black pepper

   4 teaspoons organic extra-virgin olive oil

   ¼ cup lemon juice

   1 cup white wine

   Marinate salmon with wine, lemon juice, Italian seasoning, Stevia, salt, pepper, and 1 teaspoon olive oil in dish. Ensure salmon
is completely coated and leave in fridge for 2 to 3 hours. Fire up
your grill, and then heat skillet with remaining olive oil. Toss garlic
and spinach together in pan, allowing spinach to wilt as desired. Set
aside. Place salmon over tinfoil onto grill, ensuring top side is completely coated. Cook with medium heat for 4 to 6 minutes, then turn,

coat the other side, and cook for another 4 to 6 minutes. Serve over the spinach. Makes 4 servings. Nutritional information: 20 grams of fat, 28 grams of protein, 2 grams of carbohydrates, 5 grams of fiber, and 300 calories.

Beef Pot Roast – *5 Carbs & 340 Calories*

3 pounds of beef chuck or brisket or other meat for pot roast (grass fed is preferable)

2 tablespoons organic virgin olive oil

1 tablespoon organic coconut oil

3 teaspoons Thicken Thin Not/Starch ®

1½ cups red wine

1 cup reduced-sodium beef broth

4 halved garlic cloves

4 pearl onions with skin removed

8 ounces baby carrots

4 turnips with skin removed

1 teaspoon thyme seasoning

½ teaspoon sage seasoning

½ teaspoon savory seasoning

¼ teaspoon rosemary seasoning

Using a small sharp knife, cut 8 small holes into pot roast, and place half a garlic clove in each. Heat olive oil in large skillet using medium heat. Cook roast until evenly brown on all sides, and then set aside.

Add coconut oil to pan, and add onions, cooking until brown. Add in Thicken Thin, stirring for 1 minute before adding beef broth and wine. Add all other herbs and seasoning, stirring until consistent. Place roast and sauce into Dutch oven, and cook on medium heat for 90 minutes. Add in vegetables, and cook for an additional 30 minutes. Makes 8 servings. Nutritional information: 20 grams of fat, 35 grams of protein, 5 grams of carbohydrates, 3 grams of fiber, and 340 calories.

Gourmet Cheeseburger Lettuce Wraps –
3 Carbs & 300 Calories

  1 pound top sirloin beef (you may substitute turkey or
     chicken)

  2 medium eggs

  ¼ cup whole wheat flour

  3 tablespoons low-carb ketchup or steak sauce

  1 tablespoon mustard seeds

  ½ cup shredded cheddar cheese (feel free to use another
     type)

  1 teaspoon garlic salt

  ¼ cup diced onions

  Fresh butter lettuce head.

In a large bowl, thoroughly mix beef, eggs, ketchup, and whole wheat flour. Then add all other ingredients. Once consistent, divide into 6 patties. Cook on grill using medium heat for 4 to 6 minutes. Turn, and heat for another 4 to 6 minutes. Place between two lettuce leaves and enjoy. Makes 6 servings. Nutritional information: 22 grams of fat, 22 grams of protein, 3 grams of carbs, 0 grams of fiber, and 300 calories.

OPTIONS: Find low-carb buns online to enjoy the genuine taste of a cheeseburger! Add bacon, avocado, or any of your other favorite cheeseburger derivations. Remember to budget your calories as needed and to stay under 30 grams of carbs maximum per day during the low-carb phase.

Bison Meat Loaf – *6 Carbs & 211 Calories*

  1 diced Roma tomato

  ¼ section elephant garlic

  1 teaspoon real salt

  ⅛ teaspoon cayenne pepper

  ¼ teaspoon dry mustard

  ½ teaspoon dried thyme

  1 egg

  ¼ whole red onion

½ teaspoon Worstershire sauce

1 pound ground bison

2 tablespoons rye flour

2 teaspoons glucomannan powder

First, preheat oven to 350 degrees. Combine all ingredients in one bowl, mix well, and place mixture into loaf-shaped baking pan. Bake uncovered for 75 minutes, ensuring no pink is at the center of the mixture. Center should be at least 160 degrees. Let sit for 5 minutes; slice and serve. Nutritional information: 9 grams of fat, 27 grams of protein, 6 grams of carbohydrates, 2 grams of fiber, and 211 calories.

Orange Roughy with Salsa – *4 Carbs & 120 Calories*

Marinated fish

1 pound orange roughy

⅓ cup organic low-sodium Tamari

Juice of one lemon

2 tablespoons grated fresh ginger

2 tablespoons fresh cilantro

Salsa

3 diced Roma tomatoes

½ clove elephant garlic, pressed

½ diced Anaheim chili pepper

½ diced small red onion

Dash cayenne pepper

Juice of ½ lemon or lime

¼ teaspoon real salt

¼ cup chopped cilantro

To make salsa, combine all ingredients, cover, and refrigerate for 12 hours or longer. Marinate fish for 2 hours or longer prior to cooking. Grill over tinfoil on medium heat for 5 to 10 minutes per side until done. Cover with salsa and serve. Makes 4 servings. Nutritional information: 1 gram of fat, 23 grams of protein, 4 grams of carbs, 1 gram of fiber, and 120 calories.

Bison or Beef Stew – *4 Carbs & 320 Calories*

 1½ - 2 pounds round steak

 1 cup chopped yam

 1 red onion, chopped

 ½ clove elephant garlic

 ½ cup water

 Dash Worstershire sauce

 Dash cayenne

 ¼ teaspoon sage

 ¼ teaspoon thyme

 ½ teaspoon glucomannan powder

 2 tablespoons extra-virgin olive oil

Using a large saucepan or Dutch oven over medium heat, brown the beef in olive oil. Add onions and sauté for 5 minutes longer. Add thyme, sage, cayenne, Worstershire sauce, and garlic before bringing to a broil. Bring heat to low, cover, and let simmer for 1 to 1½ more hours. Add yams and let simmer for 30 minutes longer or until tender. Place water in bowl, and whisk glucomannan powder slowly to avoid clumping. Continue until mixture is smooth and thick. Add to stew, stir, and cook until thickened. Add salt and pepper to taste. Makes 8 servings. Nutritional information: 15 grams of fat, 43 grams of protein, 4 grams of carbohydrates, 1 gram of fiber, and 320 calories.

Snack Recipes

Zucchini Stir Fry – *20 Carbs & 420 Calories*

 2 finely sliced green zucchini

 ½ chopped red pepper

 ½ chopped yellow pepper

 ¼ chopped onion

 ½ teaspoon garlic powder

 1 tablespoon dill

 ½ teaspoon pepper

2 tablespoons extra-virgin coconut oil

3 ounces of grilled chicken

2 ounces crumbled goat cheese

2 Mission Carb Balance Whole Wheat Tortillas

(Large Burrito Size)

Melt coconut oil on skillet set at medium heat, ensuring entire bottom is coated. Heat zucchini, peppers, onion, and chicken for 8 minutes or until chicken is browned. Stir in spices and cheese until melted. Set aside and let cool for 5 minutes. Heat tortillas for 30 seconds, add fillings, wrap, and serve. Makes two servings. Nutritional information: 25 grams of fat, 30 grams of protein, 20 grams of carbohydrates, 27 grams of fiber, and 420 calories. NOTE: This recipe can be made lower carb and calorie by omitting the tortillas.

Low-Carb Quesadillas – *9 Carbs & 230 Calories*

2 Mission Hills Carb Controlled Whole Wheat Tortillas (4

grams of carbs each)

2 ounces low-fat or regular shredded Mexican blend cheese

Place cheese between two tortillas on low heat until cheese is melted. Cut into fourths and enjoy. Makes one serving. Nutritional information: 12 grams of fat (18 if using full-fat cheese), 20 grams of protein, 9 grams of carbs, 16 grams of fiber, 230 calories (280 if using full-fat cheese).

Cottage Cheese and Nuts – *7 Carbs & 290 Calories*

½ cup organic non-fat cottage cheese

¼ cup nuts (almonds, macadamias, or walnuts recommended)

½ teaspoon glucomannan

½ scoop vanilla protein powder

2 teaspoons organic vanilla extract (only ingredient on label is vanilla)

Stevia to taste

Water to desired thickness (glucomannan and protein

powder will make the cottage cheese too dense without adding water—substitute half-and-half or heavy cream if you can afford the calories, or use less protein powder)

Mix ingredients together in a bowl. Add water and Stevia to achieve desired thickness and consistency. Makes 1 serving. Nutritional information (using almonds): 15 grams of fat, 31 grams of protein, 7 grams of carbs, 5 grams of fiber, and 290 calories.

Lox and Cream Cheese – *1 Carb & 210 Calories*

10 ounces lox

5 ounces cream cheese

Wrap 1 ounce of cream cheese between 2 ounces of lox and enjoy. Makes 5 servings. Nutritional information: 15 grams of fat, 15 grams of protein, 1 gram of carbohydrate, 0 grams of fiber, and 200 calories.

Turkey and Swiss Wraps – *9 Carbs & 360 Calories*

2 Mission Hills Carb Controlled Whole Wheat Tortillas (4 grams of carbs each)

2 Swiss cheese slices

2 ounces sliced turkey

1/2 teaspoon sugar-free mustard

Place a cheese slice and an ounce of turkey between each tortilla, fold over into a wrap, and serve. Makes one serving. Nutritional information: 20 grams of fat, 37 grams of protein, 9 grams of carbohydrates, 16 grams of fiber, and 360 calories.

Greek Yogurt and Nuts – *9 Carbs & 280 Calories*

1 cup nonfat plain Greek yogurt (it will have around 7 carbs and 20 grams of protein)

1/4 cup raw sliced almonds

1 tablespoon milled, organic flaxseeds

1/2 teaspoon glucomannan

Stevia to taste

Mix ingredients and enjoy. Makes 1 serving. Nutritional information: 16 grams of fat, 25 grams of protein, 9 grams of carbohydrates, 7 grams of fiber, and 280 calories.

Nuts and Cheese – *3 Carbs & 400 Calories*

1 ounce almonds, macadamias, or walnuts

2 ounces of any full-fat cheese

Serve and enjoy. Nutritional information (using almonds and Spanish Manchego cheese): 34 grams of fat, 20 grams of protein, 3 grams of carbohydrates, 2 grams of fiber, and 400 calories.

Zesty Italian Tomatoes – *3 Carbs & 150 Calories*

4 Roma tomatoes sliced in half

2 cups shredded Manchego cheese

Dash of Italian seasoning

Olive oil spray

Chicken bouillon

Butter spray

Add bouillon to top of tomatoes. Then add cheese, and spray with butter. Coat a pan with olive oil spray, and bake tomatoes at 400 degrees for 25 to 30 minutes or until soft. Add Italian seasoning, let cool for 5 to 10 minutes, and serve. Recipe makes 8 servings. Nutritional information: 12 grams of fat, 7 grams of protein, 3 grams of carbohydrates, 1 gram of fiber, and 150 calories.

Gourmet Low-Carb Nachos – *10 Carbs & 330 Calories*

3 cups shredded Manchego cheese

12 black olive halves

Chopped cilantro

$\frac{1}{2}$ cups sour cream

$\frac{1}{2}$ cups guacamole

2 tablespoons extra-virgin olive oil

8 small Mission Hills Low Carb Tortillas

Begin by lightly brushing the 8 tortillas with olive oil, and then stacking them on top of each other. Cut into 8 wedges, sprinkle with salt, and then place the chips on a single layer on a greased baking sheet. Bake at 400 degrees for 10 minutes until golden brown. Be sure to flip tortillas half-way through. Remove chips and pat down with paper towels. Place chips on a pan that can double as serving dish, and bring oven heat down to 350 degrees. Cover chips with cheese, and bake for 10 minutes until melted. Remove chips with melted cheese, and add guacamole, sour cream, olives, and salsa. Sprinkle the top with cilantro and serve. Recipe makes 5 servings. Nutritional information: 24 grams of fat, 19 grams of protein, 10 grams of carbohydrates, 14 grams of fiber, and 332 calories.

Low-Carb Enchiladas – *8 Carbs & 440 Calories*

For the shell

16 Mission Carb Balance Whole Wheat Tortillas (Small Fajita)

For the filling

2 pounds chopped chicken breast

3 chopped heads of broccoli

1 packet of low-sodium taco seasoning

1 small onion

2 garlic cloves

8 cups of pepper Jack cheese

2 tablespoons extra-virgin olive oil

For the sauce

1 stick of butter

1 large can of green enchilada sauce

¼ cup of water

3 tablespoons of heavy cream (10 grams of fat)

2 teaspoons of glucomannan powder

½ cup Jack cheese

To make the filling, pour olive oil in a pan. Sauté chopped garlic and onion. Once they are cooked a little, add the chicken, letting cook completely. Stir in chopped broccoli and taco seasoning. Broccoli doesn't have to be cooked all the way since the enchiladas will be baked in the oven.

To make the sauce, begin by making a low-carb roux. Melt butter in pan, and then slowly whisk glucomannan powder a little at a time to avoid clumping. Powder will expand in size over 5 minutes, replacing the need for flour. Add green enchilada sauce, and stir until it thickens. Stir in cream, water, and cheese, until well mixed.

To make the enchilada, fill each tortilla with broccoli and chicken mixture and cheese, and roll. Coat a baking pan with olive oil spray and line the enchiladas inside. Pour sauce over the enchiladas and cover with remaining cheese and green enchilada sauce. Bake for 25-30 minutes at 350 degrees and enjoy! Makes 16 servings. Nutritional information: 31 grams of fat, 31 grams of protein, 8 grams of carbs, 8 grams of fiber, and 440 calories. Special thanks to my friend Sheetal Parr for the recipe.

Low-Carb Pizza – *3 Carbs & 270 Calories*

Crust

1½ cups milled flaxseeds

1 teaspoon sea salt

2 teaspoon baking powder

1 teaspoon oregano

¼ teaspoon Stevia

3 eggs

3 tablespoons extra-virgin unrefined olive oil

½ cup water

Suggested Toppings

¼ cup thinly sliced bell peppers

¼ cup thinly sliced mushrooms

¼ cup diced olives

¼ cup chopped onion

½ cup shredded whole milk mozzarella cheese

½ cup shredded Parmesan cheese

½ cup shredded provolone cheese

½ cup Bella Vita Low Carb Pasta Sauce, Tomato
  Basil Style

To make the crust, add flaxseeds, oregano, Stevia, baking powder, and salt to eggs, oil, and water. Mix thoroughly and let sit for 5 to 10 minutes to thicken. Spread on greased pizza pan, and bake for 15 to 20 minutes.

Remove pizza crust, and spread on pasta sauce. Cover with cheese, and top with other ingredients. Place pizza back on greased pan and bake at 450 degrees for 8 minutes. Let cool for 5-10 minutes. Makes 8 servings. Nutritional information: 24 grams of fat, 11 grams of protein, 3 grams of carbs, 7 grams of fiber, and 270 calories.

Egg Recipes

Bacon and Cheese Frittata - *7 Carbs & 360 Calories*

¾ cup shredded Gouda cheese

½ cup heavy cream

10 ounces yellow zucchini

10 ounces broccoli

½ cup diced onion

6 large omega-3 fortified eggs

½ teaspoon salt

¼ teaspoon pepper

5 slices nitrate-free bacon

Heat oven to 350 degrees, and coat pan with organic coconut oil (you may use butter but coconut oil offers greater health benefits and fat loss). Heat bacon and onions in large skillet until bacon is crisp and onions have some brown on them. Drain fat and finely chop. Combine all other ingredients in large bowl and stir. Add in bacon and onions. When ready, pour all ingredients into pan, and bake for approximately 75 minutes. Let cool 5 to 10 minutes before serving. Makes 8 servings. Nutritional information:

28 grams of fat, 20 grams of protein, 7 grams of carbs, 3 grams of fiber, and 360 calories.

Cheese Omelet – *3 Carbs & 370 Calories*

3 medium free-range eggs

½ teaspoon glucomannan powder

2 ounces reduced-fat shredded cheese

Minced red and green peppers, onions, or any other de
   sired vegetables (optional)

Salt and pepper to taste

1 tablespoon of half-and-half

Organic coconut oil (to cook with)

Whisk eggs, vegetables, salt, pepper, and half-and-half in bowl. Slowly stir in glucomannan to avoid clumping. Coat pan on medium heat with coconut oil. Let vegetables simmer, and then remove from pan. Pour mixture from bowl and vegetables to pan and cook on medium low. Add in cheese before eggs dry. Cook to desired dryness, fold, and enjoy. Makes 1 serving. Nutritional information (plain, without added vegetables): 25 grams of fat, 34 grams of protein, 3 grams of carbohydrates, 2.5 grams of fiber, and 370 calories.

Havarti and Bacon Omelet – *3 Carbs & 350 Calories*

4 medium free-range eggs

2 ounces shredded Havarti with dill

1 tablespoon full-fat whipped cream cheese

1 tablespoon half-and-half

2 slices nitrate-free bacon (no sugar added)

¼ cup red and green peppers

1 tablespoon organic coconut oil

½ teaspoon of glucomannan powder

Salt, pepper, and dill to taste

Whisk the eggs, half-and-half, and seasonings together in a bowl. Add the cream cheese, whisking as much as needed until it's broken up as much as possible. Slowly stir in the glucomannan powder to avoid clumping. Heat coconut oil on medium heat. Cook bacon and peppers, and set aside. Add in egg mixture, and then immediately pat down with the bottom of a spoon any clumps of cream cheese until it is all evenly melted on top of the eggs. Cook to desired level before adding in cheese, bacon, and peppers. Fold and serve. Makes 2 servings. Nutritional information: 30 grams of fat, 21 grams of protein, 3 grams of carbohydrates, 3 grams of fiber, and 350 calories.

Breakfast Burritos – *8 Carbs & 240 Calories*
2 Mission Hills Whole Wheat Low Carb Tortillas
    (should have 4 grams of carbohydrates and
    8 grams of fiber each)
2 medium free-range eggs
2 ounces low-fat shredded Mexican cheese
2 tablespoons salsa
Salt and pepper to taste
¼ cup both green and red peppers
2 chopped slices deli ham (no sugar, nitrates, or
    preservatives added)
1 tablespoon half-and-half
1 teaspoon glucomannan powder
1 tablespoon organic coconut oil (for cooking)

Whisk eggs, salt, pepper, and half-and-half in bowl. Slowly add in glucomannan powder to avoid clumping. Heat coconut oil in pan on medium heat. Sauté until ham begins to brown and vegetables lose some water. Add cheese and egg mixture, and scramble together until desired dryness is achieved. Set aside and warm tortillas on pan on low heat for 60 seconds each. Pour half of egg scramble onto each tortilla, and top with one serving of salsa each. Makes 2 servings. Nutritional information: 16 grams of fat, 16 grams of protein, 8 grams of carbs, 11 grams of fiber, and 240 calories.

Shake Recipes

NOTE: For all Shake or Pudding recipes below, you'll get a thicker consistency replacing chocolate-or vanilla-flavored Met-Rx Protein Plus for Biotest's Low Carb Metabolic Drive, or using one of each type per recipe. The quality and taste of Metabolic Drive is better in my opinion, but it's hardly noticeable when using half of each, especially when thickness is desired. Also, should you have a diabetic child, these are fantastic ways of tricking them into having a delicious and healthy dessert for breakfast, lunch, or dinner without them ever realizing they just got duped into eating something healthy. Most children don't associate chocolate and vanilla shakes with healthy!

Chocolate Shake or Pudding –
7 Carbs & 210 Calories
500 ml of crushed ice to blender

Water to 500 ml after adding ice (add more for more of a
   shake consistency instead of a pudding)

1 tablespoon of vanilla extract

3 tablespoons organic raw cocoa powder (only ingredient
   should be organic cocoa)

1 tablespoon of Carlson Lab's The Very Finest Fish Oil

(can also leave out of recipe and drink in a glass of water)

2 tablespoons milled organic flaxseeds

1 teaspoon glucomannan

2 scoops Vanilla Low Carb Metabolic Drive

Stevia to taste

Blend on medium low until smooth and creamy. Makes 2 servings. Nutritional information: 11 grams of fat, 24 grams of protein, 7 grams of carbohydrates, 10 grams of fiber, and 210 calories.

Vanilla Shake or Pudding – *4 Carbs & 190 Calories*
500 ml of crushed ice to blender

Water to 500 ml after adding ice (add more for more of a
   shake consistency instead of a pudding)

1 tablespoon of vanilla extract

1 tablespoon of Carlson Lab's The Very Finest Fish Oil
(can also leave out of recipe and drink in a glass of water)

2 tablespoons milled flaxseeds

1 teaspoon glucomannan

2 scoops Vanilla Low Carb Metabolic Drive

Stevia to taste

Blend on medium low until smooth and creamy. Makes 2 servings. Nutritional information: 9.5 grams of fat, 22 grams of protein, 4 grams of carbohydrates, 7 grams of fiber, and 190 calories.

Strawberry Shake or Pudding –
7 Carbs & 200 Calories

400 ml of crushed ice to blender

Water to 500 ml after adding ice (add more for more of a
shake consistency instead of a pudding)

1 tablespoon of vanilla extract

1 tablespoon of Carlson Lab's The Very Finest Fish Oil

(can also leave out of recipe and drink in a glass of water)

2 tablespoons milled flaxseeds

1 teaspoon glucomannan

2 scoops Strawberry or Vanilla Low Carb
Metabolic Drive

100 grams organic frozen strawberries

Stevia to taste

Blend on medium low until smooth and creamy. Slightly increase blending speed and add in strawberries one by one until completely blended. Makes 2 servings. Nutritional information: 9.5 grams of fat, 22 grams of protein, 7 grams of carbohydrates, 8 grams of fiber, and 200 calories.

Pumpkin Pie Shake or Pudding –
6 Carbs & 210 Calories

500 ml of crushed ice to blender

Water to 500 ml after adding ice (add more for more of a
shake consistency instead of a pudding)

1 tablespoon of vanilla extract

1 tablespoon of Carlson Lab's The Very Finest Fish Oil
(can also leave out of recipe and drink in a glass of water)

2 tablespoons organic milled flaxseeds

½ cup organic canned pumpkin

1 teaspoon glucomannan

2 scoops Vanilla Low Carb Metabolic Drive

Pumpkin pie spice or cinnamon to taste

Stevia to taste

Blend on medium low until smooth and creamy. Makes 2 servings. Nutritional information: 10 grams of fat, 24 grams of protein, 6 grams of carbohydrates, 10 grams of fiber, and 210 calories.

Chocolate Almond Butter Shake or Pudding – *11 Carbs & 300 Calories*

500 ml of crushed ice to blender

Water to 500 ml after adding ice (add more for more of a
shake consistency instead of a pudding)

1 tablespoon of vanilla extract

3 tablespoons of organic almond butter

3 tablespoons organic raw cocoa powder (only ingredient
should be organic cocoa)

2 tablespoons milled flaxseeds

2 teaspoons glucomannan

2 scoops Chocolate or Vanilla Low Carb Metabolic Drive

Stevia to taste

Blend on medium low until smooth and creamy. Makes 2 servings. Nutritional information: 16 grams of fat, 28 grams of protein, 11 grams of carbohydrates, 8 grams of fiber, and 300 calories.

Mocha Shake or Pudding – *8 Carbs & 230 Calories*

500 ml of crushed ice to blender

Water to 500 ml after adding ice (add more for more of a
shake consistency instead of a pudding)

1 tablespoon of vanilla extract

3 tablespoons heavy whipping cream

2 teaspoons finely ground coffee

3 tablespoons organic raw cocoa powder (only ingredient
   should be organic cocoa)

2 teaspoons glucomannan

2 scoops Vanilla Low Carb Metabolic Drive

Stevia to taste

Blend on medium low until smooth and creamy. Makes 2 servings. Nutritional information: 12 grams of fat, 24 grams of protein, 8 grams of carbohydrates, 8 grams of fiber, and 230 calories.

Chocolate Coconut Shake or Pudding –
7 Carbs & 280 Calories

500 ml of crushed ice to blender

Water to 500 ml after adding ice (add more for more of a
   shake consistency instead of a pudding)

1 tablespoon of vanilla extract

2 tablespoons organic coconut oil

3 tablespoons organic raw cocoa powder (only ingredient
   should be organic cocoa)

2 teaspoons glucomannan

2 scoops Chocolate or Vanilla Low Carb Metabolic Drive

Stevia to taste

Blend on medium low until smooth and creamy. Makes 2 servings. Nutritional information: 17 grams of fat, 24 grams of protein, 7 grams of carbohydrates, 8 grams of fiber, and 280 calories.

ELEVENTH PRESCRIPTION

When You Feel Like Cheating, Remember Why You Want to be Healthy

Rule Number One – Don't Suppress How Bad You Want It!

When dealing with emotional eating, the first rule is to not suppress the desire you have for that food. If it's in front of you at the kitchen, by all means look at it. Smell it if appropriate and you so desire. Let the feelings come up.

Regret builds suppression, and suppression builds irresistible desire. Irresistible desire makes you choose to do something you would have preferred not to have done.

Don't hold back. Think of everything you love about this food—the textures, the tastes, the feeling in your heart while you're feeling it on your lips—everything. You can choose at anytime to eat that food. And when you do, you must feel no regret about it.

After Feeling the Cravings, the Next Step Is Facing the Truth

To better understand why you emotionally eat, you must run through four questions twice, first from the perspective of deciding to eat whatever you are tempted to eat, and secondly from the perspective of eating healthy food in healthy portions. The questions are designed to help you understand four different aspects of your cravings.

Beliefs: What someone *believes is the value of eating that food.*

Feelings: What someone *feels when they eat that food.*

Reasons: Why someone *thinks they should eat that food.*

Actions: What someone *does about craving that food.*

Eating Whatever in Whatever Amount

1. What do you believe is the value of eating that food?
2. How do you feel when eating that food?
3. What do you think is the reason you should eat that food?
4. What are your behaviors given this desire for this food, beyond whether or not you decide to eat it?

Eating Healthy Food in Healthy Amounts

1. What do you believe is the value of eating healthy portions of healthy food?
2. How do you feel about eating healthy portions of healthy food?
3. What do you think is the reason to eat healthy portions of healthy food?
4. What are your behaviors around eating healthy portions of healthy food, beyond whether or not you follow through?

My Answers Over That Yummy Cereal

It's Friday night, and I am exhausted from another week on a very intense commodities trading floor. I know that I need to wait until Saturday morning to start eating some carbs, but I am really edgy, and I can't get the thought of this delicious raisin and oats cereal out of my head.

The value of eating that cereal comes from needing release. After hard, exhausting work, everyone needs profound relaxation where they can forget their troubles.

While eating that cereal, I will feel that happy release from the miserable state of anxiety and exhaustion that I am in. I will also feel anxious knowing the moment will not last, and that I will need to eat more and more to keep feeling good. Afterward, I will feel gluttonous, bloated, fat, childish, and pathetic.

I think the reason to eat the cereal is because it will give me the release I need. Eating that cereal would instantly change my mood, and at this moment, I don't think that anything else in the world will.

As for my behaviors, so far I have become even more agitated and closed off, making my mood even worse.

On the flip side, the value to waiting until Saturday is that I fundamentally believe in being lean and energetic. Further, the value of not binge eating is that it proves to *me* that I have self-control—and I believe that self-control is the ultimate key to success in all aspects of life.

My emotions while eating healthy food are peaceful. End of story.

I think eating well and getting to bed will alleviate my mood better than a big binge. I am tired, so I need to sleep.

My actions are to write down in my journal everything I've eaten to motivate me to stay the course. I will also finish up everything I need to do to get to bed in time.

I wish I could tell you this moment is really easy. The truth is the one that wins is the one that you feel more. When I am bored out of my mind at work on a Friday afternoon, exhausted from another long week, and I'm not in contact with my values, my feelings and thoughts are directed toward my fatigue, anxiety, and boredom, and my behaviors can easily fall back into the old familiar pattern of emotional eating, Even in this environment, where I am numb of feeling, dull of senses, and empty inside, if I can remember my values, my feelings and thoughts, I can take the right action. If I don't do that, my actions are like leaves blowing in the wind, driven by a random force to the most familiar place.

If You're Having Trouble Deciding...

No one is telling you that you can't eat that food. You can have that food at any time. It is a choice. However, you've also made other choices. Let all the feelings about that food come up.

Think about the food when you see it. Savor it. Smell it. Admire it. Don't let the temptation build. Feel all the desire you have for that delight. What is the food doing for you? How does it make you feel? What do you think it will do for you if you eat it?

What about eating your regular healthy meal? What value does that have for you? How do you feel when you eat it? What do you think it will do for you instead?

> You don't emotionally eat because you feel things too much. You emotionally eat because you don't feel enough.

Why do you want to eat that food so much? Beyond the way it tastes, why do you want to go after it again, and again, and again? Why do you want it even after you need to loosen your belt, or even take your pants off? Why do you want it while in a food coma? These feelings are not likely to be nearly as pleasurable as the emotions around eating the food itself. Feel these feelings as well. Feel why you want as much as you do, as often as you do.

Be honest with yourself. Behind the painful reason is another more profound, freeing, more beautiful truth to be found. Staring you in the face is the very reason you overeat, and at the same time, the reason not to.

If the answer was because you were so bored talking to your family, might you really prefer a better relationship with your family, or to not be there at all? Might you prefer to relate to them in a completely different way, or to not relate to them at all? Either might be correct, but they are the reason you are overeating.

If you grabbed all the Hershey miniatures from the jar in the kitchen at work, did you do that because you didn't want to be at work then? Might you want a different job, or more help, or better hours?

If you ate ice cream after a breakup, would you have liked to have stayed in that relationship?

The answer to all these questions is "*Of course!*" So feel how bored you are—with your relatives. Feel how tired you are at work. Feel how much you love and miss that person. Feel it all, and if you still want to overeat, you are perfectly free to do so.

However, also feel how much you also want other things, things that might conflict with the choice to overeat.

> **Your choice to overeat is like currency, and it's your money to spend on whatever you want.**

It's as if you have $1,000 of play money, and you see two things you really like. You admire both options independently. You dream about what it would be like to have either. But in the end, you can choose only one, so you make your purchase, and feel happy with the choice you made. It's the same with choosing to eat something, no matter what it is, and no matter how much or how little of it there is. Ultimately, there is no wrong choice—only wanting something else more *at that time.*

Feel how much you want to be lean if that's it. Feel how much you want to respect yourself more if that's it. Feel how much you want to see your abs if that's it. Whatever it is, whatever the real reason you want to lose weight and be healthier is, feel it. Now make an informed decision, be happy with it, know you can always make the opposite decision the next time around, and live without regret.

Now ask yourself which you would choose—these reasons for eating, or other reasons for abstaining *this time*—because you can always go back. You always have the choice to eat it. And there can be no regrets should you choose to do so. Be aware of what you are choosing, know what you are giving up when you do, and be happy with your decision no matter what.

Going from Emotional Eating to Emotionally Aware Eating

1. Know that you can have whatever food you want at any time.
2. Don't block or withhold any thoughts about that food. Savor it, smell it, and remember how good it tastes.
3. At this point, ask the four questions, declaring your values, emotions, reasons, and behaviors toward eating that other food in whatever amount you want.
4. Ask the four questions again, this time declaring your values, emotions, reasons, and behaviors toward eating healthy food in healthy portions.
5. Now decide without guilt if you would rather eat that food, or stay the course with your healthy eating. More important, you must be completely comfortable with either choice.

Remember Not to Suppress Your Feelings for That "Forbidden Food"

Allow the feelings when confronted. Don't run from the temptation. Don't berate yourself. Don't feel guilty. Feel everything you feel about that food. Smell the smells. Savor the feeling. Allow it all to come in. Do not fight the sensations. You don't need to avoid tempting environments. You don't need to stay out of the candy section at the grocery store.

How to Choose Whether or Not to Act on It

You now have authentic reasons why you want to lose weight and control your diabetes. When you are confronted with the choice of eating something that will harm the choice to be healthy, you must now decide between the two. It is up to you. There should be no guilt or shame in the decision. Know that it is a choice, and make it.

TWELFTH PRESCRIPTION

Make a Plan, Write It Down, and Follow Through

*T*his is the Prescription where you just start. So many self-help books are read, the readers are inspired, but there is no follow-through. This is your life we're talking about. That cannot happen. So in the final Prescription, fill out your starting blood work numbers, fill in your starting weight, fill out your diet journal, and track your fat-loss progress. You'll see an example of a menu and how to schedule your time to exercise. You'll calculate how many calories you need every day, down to the number of grams of fat, protein, carbs, and fiber. Then, you'll create a meal plan around it. Then, you'll figure out what to do when stress and time restraints blow that plan to hell. That's it. There is no new information here. And I have made it simple to do. This is just a "do it" chapter. So let's do it.

Fill Out Your Blood Work Before Starting

Date: _____

hA1c: _____

Fasting Blood Sugar: _____

Starting Weight: _____

High-End Average Postprandial: _____

Blood Pressure: _____

HDL: _____

LDL: _____

VLDL: _____

Other Values (Kidneys, Thyroid, etc.): _____

Other Values (Kidneys, Thyroid, etc.): _____

Other Values (Kidneys, Thyroid, etc.): _____

Keep a Diet Journal

The final Prescription is about three virtues: knowledge, awareness, and accountability. Knowledge begets awareness, and awareness keeps you accountable. Diets don't usually fail because of lack of knowledge; they fail due to lack of application of knowledge. If you don't know right now what you're having for breakfast tomorrow, it's highly unlikely to be the best decision for you. That's why a journal keeps you on track. It keeps you aware of what you've done, and accountable for it. It lets you know where you're going and where you've been. To lose weight, those are the two most important pieces of information you can possibly have. You gain weight little by little because *you were never aware* that you were gaining weight little by little. A journal doesn't allow that. It forces you to know exactly what you've done to your body, whether that is good or bad. Knowledge of what makes you gain or lose fat is second only to awareness of what you're putting in your mouth.

A recent study done at Kaiser Permanente on 1,700 participants found that those who wrote down every calorie they ate in a journal lost twice as much weight or more than those who did not. There aren't even any pills on the market that can double your weight loss! Is it that hard to write stuff down now that you know it makes a difference?

Knowing what you'll do and writing it down is 50% of success. The next 25% is doing it, and the last 25% is adjusting your plan to make it better next time. Seventy-five percent of your fat loss success comes from planning, so if you think you can just eat, you'll only be 25% as successful as if you had written it down beforehand. This is the value of awareness and accountability. Turn to the Appendix and take a look at the sample journal I've included. For your convenience, a downloadable version of this journal page is available on my website, http://www.TheNewDiabetesPrescription.com. Make copies and fill it out each day. Once you do, you'll be able to learn some things about your cravings and appetite. List all caffeinated beverages and alcohol you drink, and note when you're hungry. Note the time between meals, and when you're hungry. You want this awareness.

Mark your blood sugar readings, and the times and amounts of all medications. Are your numbers outside the desired range? Are you going too low or too high during and after exercise? Have you noticed more lows even twenty-four hours after exercise?

Even When You Totally Screw Up, Write It Down

If you don't, it defeats the purpose of the journal. The purpose is to start associating cause and effect. You want to write down that a 4,000 calorie midnight cookie raid made you gain three pounds, and shot your blood sugar into the 300s. How else are you going to know the effect of that on your weight and health? Hiding it by not writing it down really doesn't work. Think about it. That's what you've always done in the past, and it's never made you face that you have a problem. That's the power of writing. If it's written down, it becomes real, and you have to deal with it.

Analyze What You've Written

Note the time and portion-size differences between each meal. This is where you analyze what you've written and reflect on it. Did you eat too little earlier, and find yourself eating a lot two hours later? Did you find that a large breakfast left you barely hungry for most of the day?

How do you feel ninety minutes after your meal? Are you energized? Are you brain fogged? Can you concentrate? Are you hungry or full?

How under stress are you? How much sleep did you get? Always record this – you'll be surprised how your appetite and cravings go up the less sleep you have. Is either work or home a stress zone right at the moment?

Take Your Measurements Once a Week After Potty and Before Breakfast

Note that you're supposed to take your measurements with a tape measure once a week. This is vital to progress and sanity. Oftentimes, the loss in inches will let you know if you're losing fat better than the scale. You can also check your body fat with a pair of body fat calipers if you wish. The choice is yours, so long as you're using one of these two methods, and not just the scale.

Now evaluate your progress. Is the scale going down? If not, are your treats causing you fat gain? Are they too great in size or frequency? What are you going to do about it?

Also, how do your clothes fit? Men, is your stomach smaller? Women, are your hips, butt, and thighs smaller? Do you see more tone?

What did you do differently on weeks where it went down instead of up? Remember that lower body fat at the same weight will always make you look leaner than lower weight at the same body fat, despite what a fashion magazine says – I put it that way because women have been lied to more often in this regard than men.

Place Morning Weight Reading in Each Box, and Measure Inches Lost Once a Week

	DAY 1	DAY 2	DAY 3	DAY 4	DAY 5	DAY 6	DAY 7	Total Pounds Lost Starting Weight ___	Total Inches Lost Starting Inches ___
WEEK 1									
WEEK 2									
WEEK 3									
WEEK 4									
WEEK 5									
WEEK 6									
WEEK 7									
WEEK 8									

There Are Other Ways to Measure Progress Besides Fat Loss and Lower Blood Sugar!

How are your eating habits progressing? Are you experiencing fewer cravings and more energy? Are you drinking less? Are you bingeing less or at all? Are you eating fewer desserts? Are you picking at sweets less? Are you able to handle stress better? Are you keeping up with your eating and exercise habits in the wake of stress or another adversary? This is all progress! Celebrate these minor victories, because you've undertaken a very long journey. You need these other forms of progress to stay motivated. When it seems like nothing is happening, notice these little things. It will keep you going!

It's Now Time to Create Your Diet

At some point in every diet book, the reader will say, "enough already – just tell me what to eat!" See the following pages for the answer – two weeks of a low-carb diet with an appropriate carb load. Mind you the calories are not appropriate for everyone – too much for some, too little for others. But the theme is dead-on for how any diabetic who wants to lose weight and control their disease should eat.

- There's plenty of eggs, fish, flax, and olive oil.
- There are five to six feedings per day every two to three hours.
- Tea and water are the two most common drinks.
- Fat, fiber, and protein are prominent in nearly every meal.
- Supplements that help with weight loss, blood sugar, cholesterol, blood pressure, and other complications are prevalent.

And on the higher-carb days…

- Keep your total calories moderate.
- You have more than your body weight in carbs, but not much more.
- You get all of those carbs from quality sources. Nothing is refined.
- You get at least 30% of your calories from fat.
- You have the greatest number of carbs first thing in the morning.
- You still eat five or six times per day, once every two to three hours.
- You still have fat, fiber, and protein at every meal to keep blood sugar down, including fat from fish and flax.
- Be sure to have the lowest fat, highest in sugar meal right after exercise, when the sugar is needed.

NOTE: The carbs are slightly less than thirty grams on most days so you can add a few from your own choices. As I mentioned already, the calories may not be appropriate for you since this is an example for everyone. That's **OK**. Just increase or decrease the recipes (except the NDP shakes) to meet your caloric requirements. The idea here is to teach you how to eat so you can burn the fat and kill the killer.

Have Water & Green Tea with Meals and Stress Buster as Needed!						

Day 1: 1,670 Calories & 20 Carbohydrates						
Meal 1	**Meal 2**	**Meal 3**	**Meal 4**	**Meal 5**	**Meal 6**	**Bedtime**
Cheese Omelet: 3 Carbs & 370 Calories	NDP Vanilla Super Shake: 2 Carbs & 240 Calories	Chef Salad with 2 tbls. Low-Carb Italian Dressing: 3 Carbs & 310 Calories	NDP Vanilla Super Shake: 2 Carbs & 240 Calories	Gourmet Cheeseburger Lettuce Wraps: 3 Carbs & 300 Calories	Chocolate Shake: 7 Carbs & 210 Calories	Have 45 to 60 Minutes Before Bed - Double If Needed
1,000 mg Taurine	2 CLA, 2 GLA	1,000 mg Taurine	2 CLA, 2 GLA	1,000 mg Taurine	1,000 mg Magnesium	0.5 mg Melatonin
300 mg Pantethine	2,000 mg Carnitine	300 mg Pantethine	2,000 mg Carnitine	300 mg Pantethine	200 mg B_6	100 mg 5-HTP
Multivitamin	100 mg CoQ10	15 mg Biotin	100 mg CoQ10	1,500 mg Inositol	4 Billion Cells Beneficial Bacteria	100 mg Theanine
Vitamin C	300 mg ALA	4,000 IU Vit. D	300 mg ALA			

Day 2: 1,820 Calories & 22 Carbohydrates						
Meal 1	**Meal 2**	**Meal 3**	**Meal 4**	**Meal 5**	**Meal 6**	**Bedtime**
Havarti & Bacon Omelet: 3 Carbs & 350 Calories	NDP Mocha Super Shake: 5 Carbs & 290 Calories	Spinach Salad with 2 tbls. Low-Carb Greek Dressing: 3 Carbs & 350 Calories	NDP Mocha Super Shake: 5 Carbs & 290 Calories	Pot Roast: 5 Carbs & 340 Calories	Lox & Cream Cheese: 1 Carb & 200 Calories	Have 45 to 60 Minutes Before Bed - Double If Needed
1,000 mg Taurine	2 CLA, 2 GLA	1,000 mg Taurine	2 CLA, 2 GLA	1,000 mg Taurine	1,000 mg Magnesium	0.5 mg Melatonin
300 mg Pantethine	2,000 mg Carnitine	300 mg Pantethine	2,000 mg Carnitine	300 mg Pantethine	200 mg B_6	100 mg 5-HTP
Multivitamin	100 mg CoQ10	15 mg Biotin	100 mg CoQ10	1,500 mg Inositol	4 Billion Cells Beneficial Bacteria	100 mg Theanine
Vitamin C	300 mg ALA	4,000 IU Vit. D	300 mg ALA			

Day 3: 1,630 Calories & 21 Carbohydrates						
Meal 1	**Meal 2**	**Meal 3**	**Meal 4**	**Meal 5**	**Meal 6**	**Bedtime**
Cheese Omelet: 3 Carbs & 370 Calories	NDP Strawberry Super Shake: 5 Carbs & 250 Calories	Chicken Caesar Salad with 2 tbls. Low-Carb Caesar Dressing: 3 Carbs & 310 Calories	NDP Strawberry Super Shake: 5 Carbs & 250 Calories	Grilled Salmon with Garlic Spinach: 2 Carbs & 300 Calories	Zesty Italian Tomatoes: 3 Carbs & 150 Calories	Have 45 to 60 Minutes Before Bed - Double If Needed
1,000 mg Taurine	2 CLA, 2 GLA	1,000 mg Taurine	2 CLA, 2 GLA	1,000 mg Taurine	1,000 mg Magnesium	0.5 mg Melatonin
300 mg Pantethine	2,000 mg Carnitine	300 mg Pantethine	2,000 mg Carnitine	300 mg Pantethine	200 mg B_6	100 mg 5-HTP
Multivitamin	100 mg CoQ10	15 mg Biotin	100 mg CoQ10	1,500 mg Inositol	4 Billion Cells Beneficial Bacteria	100 mg Theanine
Vitamin C	300 mg ALA	4,000 IU Vit. D	300 mg ALA			

Day 4: 1,760 Calories & 23 Carbohydrates

Meal 1	Meal 2	Meal 3	Meal 4	Meal 5	Meal 6	Bedtime
Havarti & Bacon Omelet: 3 Carbs & 350 Calories	NDP Chocolate Super Shake: 5 Carbs & 290 Calories	Chef Salad with 2 tbls. Low-Carb Italian Dressing: 3 Carbs & 310 Calories	NDP Chocolate Super Shake: 5 Carbs & 290 Calories	Bison or Beef Stew: 4 Carbs & 320 Calories	Low-Carb Ham & Cheese Sandwich: 3 Carbs & 200 Calories	Have 45 to 60 Minutes Before Bed - Double If Needed
1,000 mg Taurine	2 CLA, 2 GLA	1,000 mg Taurine	2 CLA, 2 GLA	1,000 mg Taurine	1,000 mg Magnesium	0.5 mg Melatonin
300 mg Pantethine	2,000 mg Carnitine	300 mg Pantethine	2,000 mg Carnitine	300 mg Pantethine	200 mg B_6	100 mg 5-HTP
Multivitamin	100 mg CoQ10	15 mg Biotin	100 mg CoQ10	1,500 mg Inositol	4 Billion Cells Beneficial Bacteria	100 mg Theanine
Vitamin C	300 mg ALA	4,000 IU Vit. D	300 mg ALA			

Day 5: 1,700 Calories & 24 Carbohydrates

Meal 1	Meal 2	Meal 3	Meal 4	Meal 5	Meal 6	Bedtime
Cheese Omelet: 3 Carbs & 370 Calories	NDP Pumpkin Super Shake: 4 Carbs & 250 Calories	Spinach Salad with 2 tbls. Low-Carb Greek Dressing: 3 Carbs & 350 Calories	NDP Pumpkin Super Shake: 4 Carbs & 250 Calories	Low-Carb Pizza: 3 Carbs & 270 Calories	Chocolate Shake: 7 Carbs & 210 Calories	Have 45 to 60 Minutes Before Bed - Double If Needed
1,000 mg Taurine	2 CLA, 2 GLA	1,000 mg Taurine	2 CLA, 2 GLA	1,000 mg Taurine	1,000 mg Magnesium	0.5 mg Melatonin
300 mg Pantethine	2,000 mg Carnitine	300 mg Pantethine	2,000 mg Carnitine	300 mg Pantethine	200 mg B_6	100 mg 5-HTP
Multivitamin	100 mg CoQ10	15 mg Biotin	100 mg CoQ10	1,500 mg Inositol	4 Billion Cells Beneficial Bacteria	100 mg Theanine
Vitamin C	300 mg ALA	4,000 IU Vit. D	300 mg ALA			

Day 6: 1,570 Calories & 30 Carbohydrates

Meal 1	Meal 2	Meal 3	Meal 4	Meal 5	Meal 6	Bedtime
Breakfast Burritos: 8 Carbs & 240 Calories	NDP Mocha Super Shake: 5 Carbs & 290 Calories	Chicken Caesar Salad with 2 tbls. Low-Carb Caesar Dressing: 3 Carbs & 310 Calories	NDP Mocha Super Shake: 5 Carbs & 290 Calories	2 Servings Orange Roughy with Salsa: 8 Carbs & 240 Calories	Lox & Cream Cheese: 1 Carb & 200 Calories	Have 45 to 60 Minutes Before Bed - Double If Needed
1,000 mg Taurine	2 CLA, 2 GLA	1,000 mg Taurine	2 CLA, 2 GLA	1,000 mg Taurine	1,000 mg Magnesium	0.5 mg Melatonin
300 mg Pantethine	2,000 mg Carnitine	300 mg Pantethine	2,000 mg Carnitine	300 mg Pantethine	200 mg B_6	100 mg 5-HTP
Multivitamin	100 mg CoQ10	15 mg Biotin	100 mg CoQ10	1,500 mg Inositol	4 Billion Cells Beneficial Bacteria	100 mg Theanine
Vitamin C	300 mg ALA	4,000 IU Vit. D	300 mg ALA			

Day 7: 1,560 Calories & 33 Carbohydrates

Meal 1	Meal 2	Meal 3	Meal 4	Meal 5	Meal 6	Bedtime
Bacon & Cheese Frittata: 7 Carbs & 360 Calories	NDP Strawberry Super Shake: 5 Carbs & 250 Calories	Low-Carb Grilled Cheese Sandwich: 3 Carbs & 270 Calories	NDP Strawberry Super Shake: 5 Carbs & 250 Calories	2 Servings Bison Chili: 10 Carbs & 280 Calories	Zesty Italian Tomatoes: 3 Carbs & 150 Calories	Have 45 to 60 Minutes Before Bed - Double If Needed
1,000 mg Taurine	2 CLA, 2 GLA	1,000 mg Taurine	2 CLA, 2 GLA	1,000 mg Taurine	1,000 mg Magnesium	0.5 mg Melatonin
300 mg Pantethine	2,000 mg Carnitine	300 mg Pantethine	2,000 mg Carnitine	300 mg Pantethine	200 mg B$_6$	100 mg 5-HTP
Multivitamin	100 mg CoQ10	15mg Biotin	100 mg CoQ10	1,500 mg Inositol	4 Billion Cells Beneficial Bacteria	100 mg Theanine
Vitamin C	300 mg ALA	4,000 IU Vit. D	300 mg ALA			

Day 8: 1,670 Calories & 20 Carbohydrates

Meal 1	Meal 2	Meal 3	Meal 4	Meal 5	Meal 6	Bedtime
Cheese Omelet: 3 Carbs & 370 Calories	NDP Vanilla Super Shake: 2 Carbs & 240 Calories	Chef Salad with 2 tbls. Low-Carb Italian Dressing: 3 Carbs & 310 Calories	NDP Vanilla Super Shake: 2 Carbs & 240 Calories	Gourmet Cheeseburger Lettuce Wraps: 3 Carbs & 300 Calories	Chocolate Shake: 7 Carbs & 210 Calories	Have 45 to 60 Minutes Before Bed - Double If Needed
1,000 mg Taurine	2 CLA, 2 GLA	1,000 mg Taurine	2 CLA, 2 GLA	1,000 mg Taurine	1,000 mg Magnesium	0.5 mg Melatonin
300 mg Pantethine	2,000 mg Carnitine	300 mg Pantethine	2,000 mg Carnitine	300 mg Pantethine	200 mg B$_6$	100 mg 5-HTP
Multivitamin	100 mg CoQ10	15 mg Biotin	100 mg CoQ10	1,500 mg Inositol	4 Billion Cells Beneficial Bacteria	100 mg Theanine
Vitamin C	300 mg ALA	4,000 IU Vit. D	300 mg ALA			

Day 9: 1,820 Calories & 22 Carbohydrates

Meal 1	Meal 2	Meal 3	Meal 4	Meal 5	Meal 6	Bedtime
Havarti & Bacon Omelet: 3 Carbs & 350 Calories	NDP Mocha Super Shake: 5 Carbs & 290 Calories	Spinach Salad with 2 tbls. Low Carb Greek Dressing: 3 Carbs & 350 Calories	NDP Mocha Super Shake: 5 Carbs & 290 Calories	Pot Roast: 5 Carbs & 340 Calories	Lox & Cream Cheese: 1 Carb & 200 Calories	Have 45 to 60 Minutes Before Bed - Double If Needed
1,000 mg Taurine	2 CLA, 2 GLA	1,000 mg Taurine	2 CLA, 2 GLA	1,000 mg Taurine	1,000 mg Magnesium	0.5 mg Melatonin
300 mg Pantethine	2,000 mg Carnitine	300 mg Pantethine	2,000 mg Carnitine	300 mg Pantethine	200 mg B$_6$	100 mg 5-HTP
Multivitamin	100 mg CoQ10	15 mg Biotin	100 mg CoQ10	1,500 mg Inositol	4 Billion Cells Beneficial Bacteria	100 mg Theanine
Vitamin C	300 mg ALA	4,000 IU Vit. D	300 mg ALA			

Day 10: 1,630 Calories & 21 Carbohydrates

Meal 1	Meal 2	Meal 3	Meal 4	Meal 5	Meal 6	Bedtime
Cheese Omelet: 3 Carbs & 370 Calories	NDP Strawberry Super Shake: 5 Carbs & 250 Calories	Chicken Caesar Salad with 2 tbls. Caesar Dressing: 3 Carbs & 310 Calories	NDP Strawberry Super Shake: 5 Carbs & 250 Calories	Grilled Salmon with Garlic Spinach: 2 Carbs & 300 Calories	Zesty Italian Tomatoes: 3 Carbs & 150 Calories	Have 45 to 60 Minutes Before Bed - Double If Needed
1,000 mg Taurine	2 CLA, 2 GLA	1,000 mg Taurine	2 CLA, 2 GLA	1,000 mg Taurine	1,000 mg Magnesium	0.5 mg Melatonin
300 mg Pantethine	2,000 mg Carnitine	300 mg Pantethine	2,000 mg Carnitine	300 mg Pantethine	200 mg B_6	100 mg 5-HTP
Multivitamin	100 mg CoQ10	15 mg Biotin	100 mg CoQ10	1,500 mg Inositol	4 Billion Cells Beneficial Bacteria	100 mg Theanine
Vitamin C	300 mg ALA	4,000 IU Vit. D	300 mg ALA			

Day 11: 1,760 Calories & 23 Carbohydrates

Meal 1	Meal 2	Meal 3	Meal 4	Meal 5	Meal 6	Bedtime
Havarti & Bacon Omelet: 3 Carbs & 350 Calories	NDP Chocolate Super Shake: 5 Carbs & 290 Calories	Chef Salad with 2 tbls. Low-Carb Italian Dressing: 3 Carbs & 310 Calories	NDP Chocolate Super Shake: 5 Carbs & 290 Calories	Bison or Beef Stew: 4 Carbs & 320 Calories	Low-Carb Ham & Cheese Sandwich: 3 Carbs & 200 Calories	Have 45 to 60 Minutes Before Bed - Double If Needed
1,000 mg Taurine	2 CLA, 2 GLA	1,000 mg Taurine	2 CLA, 2 GLA	1,000 mg Taurine	1,000 mg Magnesium	0.5 mg Melatonin
300 mg Pantethine	2,000 mg Carnitine	300 mg Pantethine	2,000 mg Carnitine	300 mg Pantethine	200 mg B_6	100 mg 5-HTP
Multivitamin	100 mg CoQ10	15 mg Biotin	100 mg CoQ10	1,500 mg Inositol	4 Billion Cells Beneficial Bacteria	100 mg Theanine
Vitamin C	300 mg ALA	4,000 IU Vit. D	300 mg ALA			

Day 12: 1,700 Calories & 24 Carbohydrates

Meal 1	Meal 2	Meal 3	Meal 4	Meal 5	Meal 6	Bedtime
Cheese Omelet: 3 Carbs & 370 Calories	NDP Pumpkin Super Shake: 4 Carbs & 250 Calories	Spinach Salad with 2 tbls. Low Carb Greek Dressing: 3 Carbs & 350 Calories	NDP Pumpkin Super Shake: 4 Carbs & 250 Calories	Low-Carb Pizza: 3 Carbs & 270 Calories	Chocolate Shake: 7 Carbs & 210 Calories	Have 45 to 60 Minutes Before Bed - Double If Needed
1,000 mg Taurine	2 CLA, 2 GLA	1,000 mg Taurine	2 CLA, 2 GLA	1,000 mg Taurine	1,000 mg Magnesium	0.5 mg Melatonin
300 mg Pantethine	2,000 mg Carnitine	300 mg Pantethine	2,000 mg Carnitine	300 mg Pantethine	200 mg B_6	100 mg 5-HTP
Multivitamin	100 mg CoQ10	15 mg Biotin	100 mg CoQ10	1,500 mg Inositol	4 Billion Cells Beneficial Bacteria	100 mg Theanine
Vitamin C	300 mg ALA	4,000 IU Vit. D	300 mg ALA			

Day 13 (High-Carb Day): 1,845 Calories & 65 Carbohydrates						
Meal 1	**Meal 2**	**Meal 3**	**Meal 4**	**Meal 5**	**Meal 6**	**Bedtime**
Eggs, Toast, & Fruit: 40 Carbs & 485 Calories	NDP Mocha Super Shake: 5 Carbs & 290 Calories	Low-Carb Enchiladas: 8 Carbs & 440 Calories	NDP Mocha Super Shake: 5 Carbs & 290 Calories	Low-Carb Grilled Cheese Sandwich: 3 Carbs & 270 Calories	Greek Yogurt & Nuts: 9 Carbs & 200 Calories	Have 45 to 60 Minutes Before Bed - Double If Needed
1,000 mg Taurine	2 CLA, 2 GLA	1,000 mg Taurine	2 CLA, 2 GLA	1,000 mg Taurine	1,000 mg Magnesium	0.5 mg Melatonin
300 mg Pantethine	2,000 mg Carnitine	300 mg Pantethine	2,000 mg Carnitine	300 mg Pantethine	200 mg B$_6$	100 mg 5-HTP
Multivitamin	100 mg CoQ10	15 mg Biotin	100 mg CoQ10	1,500 mg Inositol	4 Billion Cells Beneficial Bacteria	100 mg Theanine
Vitamin C	300 mg ALA	4,000 IU Vit. D	300 mg ALA			

Day 14 (High-Carb Day): 1,530 Calories & 71 Carbohydrates						
Meal 1	**Meal 2**	**Meal 3**	**Meal 4**	**Meal 5**	**Meal 6**	**Bedtime**
Omega Berry Oatmeal: 31 Carbs & 380 Calories	3 Crepes: 15 Carbs & 300 Calories	Gourmet Low-Carb Nachos: 10 Carbs & 330 Calories	NDP Strawberry Super Shake: 5 Carbs & 250 Calories	Low-Carb Quesadillas: 9 Carbs & 230 Calories	Happy Diabetic Cocoa: 8 Carbs & 100 Calories	Have 45 to 60 Minutes Before Bed - Double If Needed
1,000 mg Taurine	2 CLA, 2 GLA	1,000 mg Taurine	2 CLA, 2 GLA	1,000 mg Taurine	1,000 mg Magnesium	0.5 mg Melatonin
300 mg Pantethine	2,000 mg Carnitine	300 mg Pantethine	2,000 mg Carnitine	300 mg Pantethine	200 mg B$_6$	100 mg 5-HTP
Multivitamin	100 mg CoQ10	15mg Biotin	100 mg CoQ10	1,500 mg Inositol	4 Billion Cells Beneficial Bacteria	100 mg Theanine
Vitamin C	300 mg ALA	4,000 IU Vit. D	300 mg ALA			

Take Taurine 30 Minutes Before Meals. ALA Stands for Alpha Lipoic Acid

Examples of Virtually Carb Free Foods: 1 ounce full-fat cheese (9 fat grams and 7 protein grams), 1 egg (5 fat grams and 7 protein grams), 2 tablespoons ground flaxseeds (5 grams of fat and 3 grams of protein), 3.5 ounce salmon (12 grams of fat and 22 grams of protein), 3.5 ounce marbled sirloin with fat trimmed (23 grams of fat and 28 grams of protein)

Virtually Carb-Free Vegetables: spinach, broccoli, watercress, asparagus, romaine lettuce, cucumber, pickles

Foods with Five Grams of Carbs: ½ cup Greek yogurt (20 grams of protein and fat varies), ½ cup cottage cheese (15 grams of protein and fat varies), ½ cup pumpkin (negligible fat and protein), ¼ cup mixed berries (negligible fat and protein), ½ cup strawberries (negligible fat and protein), 1 slice of low-carb bread (check label), 1 or 2 low-carb tortillas (check label), 2 low-carb Atkins Bars (only uses glycerin)

Where to Get Extra Fat If Short (Negligible Carbs and Proteins): 1 ounce cream cheese (10 fat grams), 1 ounce butter (11 fat grams), 2 tablespoons of nut butter (14 fat grams), 1 tablespoon of heavy cream (5 fat grams), 1 tablespoon olive oil (14 fat grams), 1 tablespoon fish oil (12 fat grams), 14 almonds (14 fat grams), 22 macadamias (10 fat grams), 14 walnuts (20 fat grams) 1 ounce of salami (5 fat grams), 1 avocado (20 fat grams)

Where to Get Extra Protein If Short (Negligible Fats and Carbs): 3.5 ounce skinless chicken (31 grams of protein), 1 scoop whey protein (20 grams of protein), 1 can of tuna fish in water (20 grams of protein), 2 ounces of sliced turkey (13 grams of protein), 3 ounces of top sirloin with fat trimmed (24 grams of protein)

Around 20 grams of quality carbohydrates: ½ cup old-fashioned oatmeal, 2 slices Ezekiel 4:9 Bread, 1 slice of whole grain bread, 1 whole wheat tortilla, 1 grapefruit, 1 plum, 1 large peach, 1 large apple, 1 large pear, 2 medium oranges, 2 medium tangerines, 1 medium banana, 2 cups of raspberries, 2 cups of strawberries, 1 rounded cup of blueberries, ½ cantaloupe, 1 cup plain yogurt, ½ cup of black beans, ½ cup of kidney beans, ½ cup of navy beans, ½ cup of pinto beans, ½ cup quinoa, ½ cup red potatoes, 2 cups vegetable soup, 1½ cups minestrone soup

Bad carb examples: The more eaten, the sooner you'll have to return to low-carb eating: white bread, bagels, French fries, onion rings, pizza, nachos, sushi, pancakes, waffles, doughnuts, pastries, croissants, ice cream, milk shakes, pudding, chocolate, candy bars, fruit juice, colas, cookies, cakes, etc.

You Have to Count Calories to Develop Your Intuition!

You can't survive adulthood without balancing your checkbook and staying within a budget. Likewise, you can't lose fat without knowing how many calories you burn and planning meals accordingly. They are equally important life skills. It is time to master the latter. Below, you'll determine exactly how many calories you need to lose fat, including how many grams of fat, protein, and carbs at each meal. It's all spelled out for you. All that's left is learning to count calories in your foods. Read food labels, buy a book with a calorie and macronutrient breakdown for various foods, or visit http://www.nutritiondata.com for a complete nutritional breakdown of any food. There are countless online programs now that will track your fat loss for you if you prefer. For the first six months on the NDP diet, count the number of calories in your foods. Later, just knowing what you ate and its portion sizes will tell you almost everything you need to know. Once you know both how many calories are in your food, and how many calories you need to lose weight, losing will just come down to following through on that information every day.

Calculate How Many Calories You Burn Per Day (AMR)

Men's Resting Metabolic Rate:

[4.5 x Pounds] + [16 x Inches] − [5 x Years] + 5

Women's Resting Metabolic Rate:

[4.5 x Pounds] + [16 x Inches] − [5 x Years] − 161

Your RMR Is: _____

BMI = Weight (lb) x 703 ÷ Height^2 (in^2) =:_____

If your BMI is over 35, multiply your RMR by 0.85 to get a more accurate estimate. Otherwise, your RMR is accurate as is. To find your active metabolic rate (AMR), multiply your RMR by one of the following factors based on your activity level:

1.2 to 1.3 = Couch potato with a desk job who sits most
    of the day

1.4 to 1.5 = Sitting half the day, and standing half the day

1.5 to 1.6 = Teacher, mechanic, salesperson, doctor,
    or nurse, standing most of the day

1.6 to 1.7 = Typical manual laborer who's moving around
    most of the day

1.8 to 1.9 = Very physically active job such as a dancer,
    farmer, or construction worker

1.9 to 2.0 = Extremely physically active work where you're
    on your feet and working hard all day

Your AMR Is: _____

> **You have to count calories to develop your intuition! You can't survive adulthood without balancing your checkbook and staying within a budget. Likewise, you can't lose fat without knowing how many calories you burn and planning meals accordingly. They are equally important life skills.**

Now Determine How Many Calories to Eat at Each Meal

Recommended Calories Per Meal =

AMR ÷ 6: _____ calories per all 6 meals.

Recommended Grams of Fat per Meal =

0.0111 x AMR: _____.

Recommended Grams of Protein per Meal =

0.0167 x AMR - 5: _____.

Recommended Grams of Carbohydrate per Meal: <u>5 Grams</u>

Recommended Grams of Fiber per Meal: <u>5 Grams</u>

Take your weight in pounds, and divide that number by two. You need that many ounces of water per day: _____.

NOTE: No one on earth will hit these exact numbers on all six meals every day of their lives. The idea here is to total these amounts over all six meals by the end of the day. If you're supposed to eat 1,800 calories per day, and have a 600 calorie breakfast, 500 calorie lunch, 400 calorie dinner, and 100 calorie snacks, that is perfect! Kudos to you for reaching your goal for the day! So just shoot for averages around these numbers above. They're just guidelines.

Now Choose Your Own Low-Carb Menu

Breakfast is at: _____, and consists of: _____

Snack 1 is at: _____, and consists of: _____

Lunch is at: _____, and consists of: _____

Snack 2 is at: _____, and consists of: _____

Dinner is at: _____, and consists of: _____

Snack 3 is at: _____, and consists of: _____

At First, You May Experience These Temporary Symptoms That Alleviate with 100 Mg of 5-HTP & Two Grams of Glutamine: insomnia, anxiety, light-headedness, fatigue, inability to concentrate, carb cravings, moodiness or irritability, and feeling on the edge.

Average Macronutrient Breakdown on Carb-Cycling Days

Based on my BMI from the Eighth Prescription, I am qualified to carb load every/every other weekend.

Recommended Calories Per Meal =

AMR ÷ 6: _____ calories per all 6 meals

Recommended Grams of Carbohydrate per Meal =
Body Weight ÷ 20 if BMI is 30 or more,
or Body Weight ÷ 13 if BMI is under 30: _____

Recommended Grams of Fat per Meal =
[Calories Per Meal − 4 × (Carbs Per Meal)] ÷ 13

Recommended Grams of Protein per Meal =
[Calories Per Meal − 4 × (Carbs Per Meal)] ÷ 13

Recommended Grams of Fiber per Meal: 5 Grams

Take your weight in pounds, and divide that number by two. You need that many ounces of water per day: _____.

NOTE: Again, these are just averages. In particular, you can decide if you want to get all your carbs in one meal on one day, or to spread them out little by little. It really is up to you. If you do decide to have a very high-calorie, high-carb meal, the above formulas will not work. Rather, you should take a more intuitive approach. A hot fudge sundae's impact can be blunted using nutritional supplements, exercise, and cutting carbs for the remaining meals in the day. In other words, balance the good with the bad.

Do you drink alcohol? From where will you get your two drinks *max* **per day on the weekends?** _____

Count indulgences toward total carbs!
Cut down on other meals to budget!

On Saturday, my indulgence meal will be:

_____.

On Sunday, my indulgence meal will be:

_____.

Now Choose Your Own Carb-Cycling Menu

Breakfast is at: _____, and consists of: _____

Snack 1 is at: _____, and consists of: _____

Lunch is at: _____, and consists of: _____

Snack 2 is at: _____, and consists of: _____

Dinner is at: _____, and consists of: _____

Snack 3 is at: _____, and consists of: _____

Symptoms of too many carbs, meaning time to cut carbs again: High blood sugar, fatigue, bloat, water retention, puffiness, severe carb cravings, irritability, moodiness, sleepiness, fat gain, poor concentration, mental fogginess, food coma.

Have a Plan for When It Hits the Fan

What's going to happen when the boss needs overtime, or the kids have soccer practice, and you're too tired to cook? Stress is the number one reason that a change in eating habits fails. Your new habits can't simply work in calm waters. You have to know exactly what you're going to eat when stress is at its worst. It has to be pre-determined. And it has to taste good. What foods are portable, tasty, and easily prepared?

Life will get in the way. There's no escaping it. The trick is to recognize when a situation will demand more of your time. You will then have to plan to make meals that are:

- Delicious
- Filled with enough but not too many fats, carbs, proteins, and fiber
- Easily prepared
- Portable

A protein smoothie made with natural fruit and protein powder is a perfect example. An example would be a strawberry smoothie made with a ½ cup of strawberries, 1½ scoops of protein powder, 3 tablespoons of flaxseeds, 1 teaspoon of fish oil, cinnamon, and Stevia. Such a drink has 30 grams of protein, 13 grams of fat, and 5 grams of carbohydrates. You could also grill lean beef with steamed broccoli and spinach, and drizzle in olive oil. Packing a salad made from last night's healthy leftovers would also work.

Remember: times of stress make you want to eat worse, eat a lot, and exercise less. The only difference between the lean and you is that they still eat healthily, still eat the same amounts, and still exercise the same even in times of stress. They find a way to do so regardless of what else is happening in their lives. They make no excuses. Be like them to become one of them! I wake up at 4:15 AM to exercise before arriving at work at 5:30 AM. My meals were prepped and packed the night before.

Stress will occur on _____, so I will prepare for that time.

Food will be scarce on _____, so I will prepare for that time.

Temptation will be found at _____,

so I will _____.

Hostility will be encountered at _____,

so I will _____.

I will shop for my weekly food on this day

of the week: _____.

Again, write down why you want to exercise: _____

_____

_____

Now Choose Your Times to Exercise

Go to http://www.TheNewDiabetesPrescription.com for a free copy of an exercise journal.

Weight Training Is Done Three Times per Week on Non-Consecutive Days. I choose _____, _____, & _____ as my three days to lift weights.

Cardiovascular Exercise Is Done Three Times per Week after Weight Training, or on Three Non-Weight Training Days. I choose _____, _____, & _____ as my three times to perform cardiovascular exercise.

My Own Blood Profiles After Practicing What I've Preached

Cholesterol Total (combination of HDL and LDL): 161 mg/dl

HDL (high-density lipids or good cholesterol): 89 mg/dl

LDL (low-density lipids or bad cholesterol): 72 mg/dl

Triglycerides (also called VLDL or very low-density lipids – this is a part of LDL): 42 mg/dl (my internist said this was the lowest she's seen in anyone ever)

hA1c: 4.9 – 5.1% for the past five years!

Kidneys, liver, blood pressure, and thyroid: All OK!

So despite a diet of over 60% fat, since the carbs were low and the fats were exceptional, I'm doing wonderfully! Even if you have cholesterol problems, don't be afraid of fat! Processed carbohydrates have done more to increase bad cholesterol than a filet mignon ever has!

I'll go up against any critic of low-carb diets with my blood profiles. Test me. My kidneys and liver and everything else are fine, too, according to multiple blood tests over multiple years. Behold the blood work of a thirty-two-year-old man who has been low carbing it for over seven years as of this publication. That's longer than many studies actually done with diabetics on low-carb diets! Can we bury the belief that these ways of eating are not safe?

You Now Know What You Need to Do

The idea in this book was to help you identify *what you do* that exacerbates weight gain, high blood sugar, and all the complications of diabetes – that which you do to yourself that you can change. There is a right and wrong choice among breads. There is a right and wrong choice among fats. There is a right and wrong choice among drinks. It is black and white. In the world of recovering your health, there is little room for gray.

There is so much wishy-washy advice thrown at diabetics. Everyone is afraid of giving you too many restrictions, too few choices, that they rob you of seeing what's really hurting you by making you think it's all OK. "Eat white bread in moderation," they say. How about just don't eat white bread? "Moderate your soda." How about no soda? "Get exercise in five minute bouts, and park farther away from the office." Sorry, this is just not enough. It doesn't add up.

I was not afraid to tell you what you really need to do because I've been you. I was fat, sedentary with high blood sugar for years. And now I'm not. And in this book I've shared with you how I stopped.

If you know me, you'll know I'll still have more cheesecake than I'd like at Thanksgiving. You'll see me sometimes still eat the Hershey Miniatures in the work kitchen. Too much work and too little sleep still get to me. But if you watch me over twenty-four hours for 365 days, you'll see why I've managed to keep the weight off and the blood sugar down: consistency. The 5% of screwing up I do is not beating the 95% of when I get it right with my diet and exercise.

Stay consistent.

**Be kind to yourself when you screw up.
Get up, dust yourself off, and just keep going.
Figure out what caused the binge.**

What happened that day inside of you and outside of you to spark it? There was a reason. And it will happen again. Every time you uncover one of the mechanisms that add to your overeating and undermoving, you've created a leaner future version of you. Celebrate that. Then find the next one.

I've started a club at my website, http://www.TheNewDiabetesPrescription.com, for all of you to come and get more support. There you will find my blog, exercises you can do at home, more recipes, a chat room, and one-on-one assistance if you need it. You are not alone.

This is also the first of a series of books on diabetes. If you need more help with heart attacks, strokes, pregnancies, childhood diabetes, stress, or more, it's on the way.

Please stop by my website and share your successes and failures with others. Together, we can find what works best for everyone. Your story will help others just as I hope my story has helped you. Thank you for taking the time to read it.

APPENDIX

The New Diabetes Prescription Daily Nutrition Journal				
Date ____ Body Weight____ Total Inches Lost____ Fasting Glucose____ Exercise Min.____ Sleep Hrs.____				
Time	Breakfast	Nutritional Info	Supplements & Meds	Readings
		Fat		Pre-Prandialial
Cravings		Protein		Post-Prandial
		Carbs		BP
		Fiber		Other
		Calories		Other
Time	Snack 1	Nutritional Info	Supplements & Meds	Readings
		Fat		Pre-Prandial
Cravings		Protein		Post-Prandial
		Carbs		BP
		Fiber		Other
		Calories		Other
Time	Lunch	Nutritional Info	Supplements & Meds	Readings
		Fat		Pre-Prandial
Cravings		Protein		Post-Prandial
		Carbs		BP
		Fiber		Other
		Calories		Other
Time	Snack 2	Nutritional Info	Supplements & Meds	Readings
		Fat		Pre-Prandial
Cravings		Protein		Post-Prandial
		Carbs		BP
		Fiber		Other
		Calories		Other
Time	Dinner	Nutritional Info	Supplements & Meds	Readings
		Fat		Pre-Prandial
Cravings		Protein		Post-Prandial
		Carbs		BP
		Fiber		Other
		Calories		Other
Time	Snack 3	Nutritional Info	Supplements & Meds	Readings
		Fat		Pre-Prandial
Cravings		Protein		Post-Prandial
		Carbs		BP
		Fiber		Other
		Calories		Other
Total Calories _____ Total Carbs _____ Total Fat _____ Total Protein _____ Total Fiber _____				

First Prescription:
Be Accountable and Take Control

1. National Health Institute website, http://diabetes.niddk.nih.gov/dm/ pubs/statistics/index.htm, accessed 10-11-2009.

2. Centers for Disease Control and Prevention website, "CDC's Diabetes Program-News and Information-Press Releases-October 26 2000". http://www.cdc.gov/Diabetes/news/docs/010126.htm, accessed 10-11-2009.

3. Wild S, Roglic G, Green A, Sicree R, King H, "Global Prevalence of Diabetes: Estimates for the Year 2000 and Projections for 2030," Diabetes Care 27 (5): 1047–53. doi:10.2337/diacare.27.5.1047. PMID 15111519

4. Narayan K, Boyle J, Thompson T, Sorensen S, Williamson D, "Lifetime risk for diabetes mellitus in the United States". JAMA 290 (14): 1884–90. doi:10.1001/jama.290.14.1884. PMID 14532317.

5. American Diabetes Association website, "Total Prevalence of Diabetes & Pre-diabetes". http://www.diabetes.org/diabetes-statistics/ prevalence.jsp. Accessed 10-11-2009.

6. Jellinger, Paul S. "What You Need to Know about Pre-diabetes." Power of Prevention, American College of Endocrinology. Vol. 1, issue 2, May 2009. http://www.powerofprevention.com/

7. Wilson, James L., N.D., D.C., Ph.D., Adrenal Fatigue: The 21st Century Stress Syndrome, (1st edition), Petaluma, CA: Smart Publications, 2003. PP 257-284

8. Richards, Byron J., CCN, Mastering Leptin: The Leptin Diet, Solving Obesity And Preventing Disease! (2nd edition), Minneapolis, Minnesota: Wellness Resources Books, 2002. PP 158

9. Richards, Byron J., CCN, Mastering Leptin: The Leptin Diet, Solving Obesity And Preventing Disease! (2nd edition), Minneapolis, Minnesota: Wellness Resources Books, 2002. PP 31, 41

10. DeLany, J., "Leptin hormone and other biochemical influences on systemic inflammation," J Bodyw Moy Ther. 2008 Apr:12(2):121-32

11. Gittleman, Ann Louise, M.S., C.N.S., The Fat Flush Plan, McGraw Hill, 2002. PP 36-38

12. Seematter, G., Binnert, C., Tappy, L. "Stress and metabolism," Metab Syndr Relat. Disord., 2005;3(1):8-13

13. Parker, Michelle, "How to Lose Visceral Fat," http://ezinearticles. com/?How-to-Lose-Visceral-Fat&id=657916, accessed on 06-20-2009

14. Acheson KJ, Schutz Y, Bessard T, Anantharaman K, Flatt JP, Jéquier E., "Glycogen storage capacity and de novo lipogenesis during massive carbohydrate overfeeding in man," Am Journal of Clinical Nutrition 1988 Aug;48(2):240-7.

15. Richards, Byron J., CCN, Mastering Leptin: The Leptin Diet, Solving Obesity And Preventing Disease! (2nd edition), Minneapolis, Minnesota: Wellness Resources Books, 2002. PP 119, 169-173

16. Kolaczynski JW, Ohannesian JP, Considine RV, Marco CC, Caro JF. Response of leptin to short-term and prolonged overfeeding in humans. J Clin Endocrinol Metab 1996 Nov;81(11):4162-5

17. Banks WA, Coon AB, Robinson SM, Moinuddin A, Shultz JM, Nakaoke R, Morley JE., "Triglycerides induce leptin resistance at the blood-brain barrier." Diabetes, 2004 May;53(5):1253-60.

18. Sinha MK, Caro JF., "Clinical aspects of leptin," Vitam Horm. 1998;54:1-30.

19. Vernon, M., Eberstein, J., Atkins Diabetes Revolution (1st Edition) New York: Harper Collins, 2004, Page 36.

20. Vernon, M., Eberstein, J., Atkins Diabetes Revolution (1st Edition) New York: Harper Collins, 2004, Page 37.

21. Edelman, Steven V., M.D., et al, Taking Control Of Your Diabetes (2nd Edition), Professional Communications Inc., 2001.

22. The Diabetes Control and Complications Trial Research Group, "The effect of intensive treatment of diabetes on the development and progression of long-term complications in insulin-dependent diabetes mellitus." N Engl J Med. 1993 Sep 30;329(14):977-86 PMID 8366922. Retrieved 9/19/2009.

23. UK Prospective Diabetes Study Website, http://www.dtu.ox.ac.uk/

index.php?maindoc=/ukpds/index.php, accessed 9/19/2009.

24. Reynisdottir S., Wahrenberg H., Carlström K., Rössner S., Arner P.," Catecholamine resistance in fat cells of women with upper-body obesity due to decreased expression of beta2-adrenoceptors" Diabetologia, 1994 April;37(4):428-435.

25. Forbes S, Robinson S, Parker KH, Macdonald IA, McCarthy MI, Johnston DG., "The thermic response to food is related to sensitivity to adrenaline in a group at risk for the development of type II diabetes." Eur. J. Clin. Nutr., 2009 Aug 26 PMID: 19707224.

Second Prescription:
Control Emotional Eating
to Control Your Blood Sugar

1. Richards, Byron J., CCN, Mastering Leptin: The Leptin Diet, Solving Obesity And Preventing Disease! (2nd edition), Minneapolis, Minnesota: Wellness Resources Books, 2002. Page 180

2. Richards, Byron J., CCN, Mastering Leptin: The Leptin Diet, Solving Obesity And Preventing Disease! (2nd edition), Minneapolis, Minnesota: Wellness Resources Books, 2002. Page 116, 182, 253.

3. Wurtman, R.J. and J.J., "Brain Serotonin: Carbohydrate Craving, Obesity, and Depression," Adv. Exp. Med. Biol. 398 (1996): 35-41.

4. Halford, JC, Blundell, JE, "Separate Systems for serotonin and leptin in appetite control," Ann. Med. 2000 April 32(3): 222-32.

5. Richards, Byron J., CCN, Mastering Leptin: The Leptin Diet, Solving Obesity And Preventing Disease! (2nd edition), Minneapolis, Minnesota: Wellness Resources Books, 2002. Page 158-162 & 170-172

6. Richards, Byron J., CCN, Mastering Leptin: The Leptin Diet, Solving Obesity And Preventing Disease! (2nd edition), Minneapolis, Minnesota: Wellness Resources Books, 2002. Page 160

7. Richards, Byron J., CCN, Mastering Leptin: The Leptin Diet, Solving Obesity And Preventing Disease! (2nd edition), Minneapolis, Minnesota: Wellness Resources Books, 2002. Page 169

8. Keijzers, GB, De Galan, BE, Tack CJ, Smits, P, "Caffeine can de-

crease insulin sensitivity in humans," Diabetes Care, 2002 Feb 25(2):364-9.

9. Gardner, Amanda, "Study Suggests Sugar May Be Addictive Finding might yield new insights into eating disorders, experts say," http://vsnrc.reshealth.org/yourhealth/newsarticle. cfm?articleID=622127 accessed on 12/11/2008

10. Davis, C, et. al, "Reward sensitivity and the D2 dopamine receptor gene: A case-control study of binge eating disorder." Prog Neuropsychopharmacol Biol Psychiatry. 2008 Apr 1;32(3):620-8. Epub 2007 Oct 10.

11. Wurtman R.J., Wurtman, J.J., "Brain Serotonin, Carbohydrate-Craving, Obesity, and Depression." Advanced Experimental Medical Biology 398 (1996): 35-41

12. Blum, K, et. al., "Reward Deficiency Syndrome," http://www.recoveryemporium.com/Articles/AmSci.htm, accessed on 12/11/2008.

13. N.S., "Does lack of sleep lead to diabetes?" http://findarticles.com/p/articles/mi_m1200/is_2_160/ai_77049898, accessed on 12/8/2008

14. Gittleman, Ann Louise, M.S., C.N.S., The Fat Flush Plan, McGraw Hill, 2002. PP 101

15. Jenkins, D., et al. Nibbling versus gorging: metabolic advantages of increased meal frequency. N Engl J Med 1989 321(14): 929-934.

16. Speechly, D. and Buffenstein, R. Greater appetite control associated with an increased frequency of eating in lean males. Appetite 1999 33(3): 285-297.

17. Birdsall, T.C., "5-Hydroxytryptophan: A Clinically-Effective Serotonin Precursor," Altern Med Rev 3.4 (1998): 271-80.

18. Byerley, W.F., et al., "5-Hydroxytryptophan: A Review of its Antidepressant Efficacy and Adverse Effects," J Clin Psychopharmacol 7.3 (1987) : 127-37.

19. Murray, Michael,, N.D., Pizzorno, Joseph, N.D., Encyclopedia of Natural Medicine. Prima Health, 1998. PP 390-393, 683-688

20. Ceci, F., et al., "The Effects of Oral 5-Hydroxytryptophan Administration on Feeding Behavior in Obese Adult Female Subjects," J Neural Transm 76.2 (1989): 109-17.

21. Cangiano, C., et al., "Eating Behavior and Adherence to Dieatary Prescriptions in Obese Adult Subjects treated with 5-Hydroxytrypto-phan." American Journal of Clinical Nutrition 56 (1992): 863-867

22. Lam, DD, et. al., "Serotonin 5-HT2C receptor agonist promotes hy-pophagia via downstream activation of melanocortin 4 receptors," Endocrinology 2008 Mar;149(3):1323-8. Epub 2007 Nov 26

23. Zhou, L, et. al., "Serotonin 2C receptor agonists improve type II diabetes via melanocortin-4 receptor signaling pathways," Cell Me-tab.2007 Nov;6(5):398-405.

24. Atkins, Robert C., M.D., Dr. Atkins' Vita-Nutrient Solution: Nature's Answer To Drugs, Fireside, 1999. PP 167-170

25. Atkins, Robert C., M.D., Dr. Atkins' Vita-Nutrient Solution: Nature's Answer To Drugs, Fireside, 1999. PP 304

26. Loehr, Jim, Schwartz, Tony, "The Power Of Full Engagement: Man-aging Energy, Not Time, Is the Key to High Performance and Per-sonal Renewal," Free Press, 2003.

27. Zinczzenko, David, Goulding, Matt, "The Truth About Diet Soda," http://health.yahoo.com/experts/eatthis/22630/the-truth-about-diet-soda, accessed 2-2-2009.

Third Prescription:
Change the Stress, or Change Your Response

1. Lu K, Gray M, Oliver C, Liley D, Harrison B, Bartholomeusz C, Phan K, Nathan P (2004). "The acute effects of L-theanine in com-parison with alprazolam on anticipatory anxiety in humans". Hum Psychopharmacol 19 (7): 457–65.

2. Kimura K, Ozeki M, Juneja L, Ohira H (2007). "L-Theanine re-duces psychological and physiological stress responses". Biol Psychol 74 (1): 39–45.

3. Murray, M, "L-Theanine: The Next Supplement Superstar," pub-lished www.doctormurray.com, September 20th, 2006. Accessed 7-3-2007

4. Siena, D, "The Magic of Green Tea: An Ancient Panacea for a Modern World," http: www.acupuncturetoday.com/ archives2003/

jun/06siena.html, accessed 7-5-2007

5. Richards, Byron J., CCN, Mastering Leptin: The Leptin Diet, Solving Obesity And Preventing Disease! (2nd edition), Minneapolis, Minnesota: Wellness Resources Books, 2002. PP 164

6. Dulloo, A.G., et al., "Efficacy of a Green Tea Extract Rich in Catechin Polyphenols and Caffeine in Increasing 24-h Energy Expenditure and Fat Oxidation in Humans," Amer J Clin Nutr 70.6 (1999) : 1040-5.

7. Dulloo, A.G., et al., "Green Tea and Thermogenesis: Interactions Between Catechin-Polyphenols, Caffeine and Sympathetic Activity," Int J Obes Relat Metab Disord 24.2 (2000) : 252-8.

8. Manning J, Roberts JC. "Analysis of catechin content of commercial green tea products." J Herb Pharmacother. 2003;3(3):19-32.

9. Henning SM, et al. "Catechin content of 18 teas and a green tea extract supplement correlates with the antioxidant capacity." Nutr Cancer. 2003;45(2):226-35.

10. Mowry, D,"Does Yerba Mate Contain Any Caffeine?," http://www.a1b2c3.com/drugs/yer_02.htm, Found 7-5-2007

11. Atkins, Robert C., M.D., Dr. Atkins' Vita-Nutrient Solution: Nature's Answer To Drugs, Fireside, 1999. PP 172-174

12. Hitsman et. al., "Effects of acute tyrosine/phenylalanine depletion on the selective processing of smoking-related cues and the relative value of cigarettes in smokers," Psychopharmacology (Berl). 2008 Mar;196(4):611-21 Epub 2007 Nov 25.

13. Richards, Byron J., CCN, Mastering Leptin: The Leptin Diet, Solving Obesity And Preventing Disease! (2nd edition), Minneapolis, Minnesota: Wellness Resources Books, 2002. PP 170-171, 177

14. Wilson, James L., N.D., D.C., Ph.D., Adrenal Fatigue: The 21st Century Stress Syndrome, (1st edition), Petaluma, CA: Smart Publications, 2003. PP 193-207

15. Atkins, Robert C., M.D., Dr. Atkins' Vita-Nutrient Solution: Nature's Answer To Drugs, Fireside, 1999. PP 253-255

16. Wilson, James L., N.D., D.C., Ph.D., Adrenal Fatigue: The 21st Century Stress Syndrome, (1st edition), Petaluma, CA: Smart Publica-

tions, 2003. PP 218-219

17. Haskell CF, Kennedy DO, Milne AL, Wesnes KA, Scholey AB (2008). "The effects of l-theanine, caffeine and their combination on cognition and mood". Biol Psychol 77 (2): 113–22.

18. Berardi et. al., "Roundtable: Caffeine", http://t-nation.com/free_online_article/ sports_ body_training_performance_interviews/caffeine_roundtable, accessed 7-3-2007

19. Bryan, J., "Psychological effects of dietary components of tea: caffeine and L-theanine," Nutr Rev. 2008 Feb;66(2):82-90

20. Nathan P, Lu K, Gray M, Oliver C (2006). "The neuropharmacology of L-theanine(N-ethyl-L-glutamine): a possible neuroprotective and cognitive enhancing agent". J Herb Pharmacother 6 (2): 21–30.

21. Chatkin, Jr, Chatkin JM, "Smoking and changes in bodyweight: can pathophysiology and genetics explain this association? (originally in Portuguese)" J Bras Pnemol., 2007 Dec;33(6):712-719

22. Davis, C, et. al. "Reward sensitivity and the D2 dopamine receptor gene: A case-control study of binge eating disorder," Prog Neuropsychopharmacol Biol Psychiatry. 2008 Apr 1;32(3):620-8. Epub 2007 Oct 10

23. Banderet, L.E., and Lieberman, H.R., "Treatment with Tyrosine, a Neurotransmitter Precursor, Reduces Environmental Stress in Humans," Brain Res Bull 22 (1989) : 759-62.

24. Deijen, J.B., et al., "Tyrosine Improves Cognitive Performance and Reduces Blood Pressure in Cadets After One week of a Combat Training Course," Brain Res Bull 48.2 (1999) : 203-9.

25. Gelenberg, A.J., et al., "Tyrosine for Depression," J Psychiatr Res 17.2 (1982-83) :175-80.

26. Gelenberg, A.J., and Gibson, C.J., "Tyrosine for the Treatment of Depression," Nutr Health 3.3 (1984) : 163-73.

27. Editors at Health Day, "Nicotine May Help Spur 'Pre-diabetes'," http://yourtotalhealth.ivillage.com/nicotine-may-help-spur-prediabetes.html?nlcid=di|06-23-2009|, accessed on 6-28-2009

Fourth Prescription:
Exercise Is the Best Medication

1. Johannsson, E., Effect of cross-reinnervation on the expression of GLUT-4 and GLUT-1 in slow and fast rat muscles. Am J Physiol. 1996 Jun;270(6 Pt 2):R1355-60.

2. Phillips, S., et al. Increments in skeletal muscle GLUT-1 and GLUT-4 after endurance training in humans. Am J Physiol. 1996 Mar;270(3 Pt 1):E456-62.

3. Whelton SP, Chin A, Xin X, He J., "Effect of aerobic exercise on blood pressure: a meta-analysis of randomized, controlled trials," Ann Intern Med. 2002 Apr 2;136(7):493-503.

4. Smutok, M., et al. (1994). Effects of exercise training modality on glucose tolerance in men with abnormal glucose regulation. Int J Sports Med 15(6): 283-289.

5. Houmard, JA., et. al., "Exercise training increases GLUT-4 protein concentration in previously sedentary middle-aged men," Am J Physiol., 1993 Jun; 264(6 Pt 1):E896-901

6. Washington Post (source not named), "As duties pile up, Obama's faith in fitness grows: President-elect cuts back on novels, watching TV but seldom skips the gym," http://www.msnbc.msn.com/id/2838463, accessed on 12-25-2008

7. Cressey, Eric, Robertson, Mike, "Magnificent Mobility: 10 Minutes To Better Flexibility, Performance, and Health," DVD by Mike Robertson and Eric Cressey, 2005.

8. Hartman, Bill, Robertson, Mike, Inside-Out: The Ultimate Upper Body Warm-Up (e-book), Bill Hartman and Mike Robertson, 2006.

9. McGill, Stuart, Ph.D., Ultimate Back Fitness And Performance (3rd Edition), Wabuno Publishers, Backfitpro Inc., 2006.

10. Tsatsouline, Pavel, Power To The People! Russian Strength Training Secrets For Every American, Dragon Door Publications Inc., 2000.

11. Tsatsouline, Pavel, Beyond Bodybuilding: Muscle And Strength Training Secrets For The Renaissance Man, Dragon Door Publications Inc., 2005.

12. Tsatsouline, Pavel, "The Russian Kettlebell Challenge, Dragon Door

Publications Inc., 2001

13. Tsatsouline, Pavel, "Enter The Kettlebell, Dragon Door Publications Inc., 2006

14. Wilmore, J.H., and Costill, D.L., Training for Sport and Activity: The Physiology Basis of the Conditioning Process, (3rd edition), Duboque, IA: Wm. C. Brown Publishers, 1988.

15. Phillips, Bill, Body for Life, 11th Vision LLC, 1999.

16. Phillips, Shawn, ABSsolution: The Practical Solution for Building Your Best Abs, High Point Media LLC, 2002.

17. Davies, Clair NCTMB, The Trigger Point Therapy Workbook: Your Self-Treatment Guide For Pain Relief, 2nd Edition, New Harbinger Publications, Inc., 2004

18. Barnard, R.J., T. Jung, S.B. Inkeles, "Diet and exercise in the treatment of NIDDM - the need for early emphasis." Diabetes Care, 17:1469-1472, 1994

Fifth Prescription:
Follow a Low-Carb Diet Most of the Time

1. Volek JS, Phinney SD, Forsythe CE, Quann EE, Wood RJ, Puglisi MJ, Kraemer WJ, Bibus DM, Fernandez ML, Feinman RD, "Carbohydrate Restriction has a More Favorable Impact on the Metabolic Syndrome than a Low Fat Diet," Lipids. 2008 Dec 12. [Epub ahead of print] PMID: 19082851 [PubMed - as supplied by publisher]

2. 2) Torres-Gonzalez M, Volek JS, Leite JO, Fraser H, Luz Fernandez M., "Carbohydrate restriction reduces lipids and inflammation and prevents atherosclerosis in Guinea pigs," J Atheroscler Thromb. 2008 Oct;15(5):235-43. PMID: 18981648 [PubMed - in process]

3. Accurso A, Bernstein RK, Dahlqvist A, Draznin B, Feinman RD, Fine EJ, Gleed A, Jacobs DB, Larson G, Lustig RH, Manninen AH, McFarlane SI, Morrison K, Nielsen JV, Ravnskov U, Roth KS, Silvestre R, Sowers JR, Sundberg R, Volek JS, Westman EC, Wood RJ, Wortman J, Vernon MC. "Dietary carbohydrate restriction in type II diabetes mellitus and metabolic syndrome: time for a critical appraisal," Nutr Metab (Lond). 2008 Apr 8;5:9. PMID: 18397522

[PubMed - in process]

4. Boden, G., Sargrad, K., Homko, C., et. al., "Effect of a Low-Carbohydrate Diet on Appetite, Blood Glucose Levels, and Insulin Resistance in Obese Patients with Type II Diabetes," Annals of Internal Medicine, 142(6), 2005, pages 403-411.

5. Buchholz AC, Schoeller DA.,"Is a calorie a calorie?" Am J Clin Nutr. 2004 May;79(5):899S-906S.

6. Feinman RD, Volek JS. "Low carbohydrate diets improve atherogenic dyslipidemia even in the absence of weight loss," Nutr Metab (Lond). 2006 Jun 21;3:24. PMID: 16790045 [PubMed]

7. Wood RJ, Volek JS, Liu Y, Shachter NS, Contois JH, Fernandez ML.,"Carbohydrate restriction alters lipoprotein metabolism by modifying VLDL, LDL, and HDL subfraction distribution and size in overweight men," J Nutr. 2006 Feb;136(2):384-9.PMID: 16424116

8. Reaven G, Backes AC, Abbasi F, Lamendola C, McLaughlin TL, Palaniappan LP. "Clinical experience with a relatively low carbohydrate, calorie-restricted diet improves insulin sensitivity and associated metabolic abnormalities in overweight, insulin resistant South Asian Indian women," Asia Pac J Clin Nutr. 2008;17(4):669-71. PMID: 19114407 [PubMed - in process]

9. Okere IC, "Low carbohydrate/high-fat diet attenuates cardiac hypertrophy, remodeling, and altered gene expression in hypertension," Hypertension 2006 Dec;48(6):111-23 Epub 2006 Oct 23

10. Duda, MK, et al, "Low Carbohydrate/high-fat diet attenuates pressure overload-induced ventricular remodeling and dysfunction," J Card Fail 2008 May;14(4):327-335 PMID: 18474346

11. Volek JS, Feinman RD., "Carbohydrate restriction improves the features of Metabolic Syndrome. Metabolic Syndrome may be defined by the response to carbohydrate restriction," Nutr Metab (Lond). 2005 Nov 16;2:31. PMID: 16288655

12. McCarger LJ, Baracos VE and Clandinin MT. Influence of dietary carbohydrate-to-fat ratio on whole body nitrogen retention and body composition in adult rats. Journal of Nutrition 1989; 119(9):1240-5

13. Layman, D., et al. (2003). A reduced ratio of dietary carbohydrate to

protein improves body composition and blood lipid profiles during weight loss in adult women. J Nutr 133(2): 411-417.

14. Volek JS, Sharman MJ, Love DM, Avery NG, Gómez AL, Scheett TP, Kraemer WJ.,"Endurance capacity and high-intensity exercise performance responses to a high fat diet," Int J Sport Nutr Exerc Metab. 2003 Dec;13(4):466-78. PMID: 14967870 [PubMed - indexed for MEDLINE]

15. Rabast U, Kasper H, Shonborn J. Comparative studies in obese subjects fed carbohydrate-restricted and high carbohydrate 1,000-calorie formula diets. Nutritional Metabolism 1978; 22(5):269-77

16. Feinman RD, Volek JS., "Carbohydrate restriction as the default treatment for type II diabetes and metabolic syndrome," Scand Cardiovasc J. 2008 Aug;42(4):256-63. PMID: 18609058 [PubMed - in process]

17. Ratliff JC, Mutungi G, Puglisi MJ, Volek JS, Fernandez ML. "Eggs modulate the inflammatory response to carbohydrate restricted diets in overweight men," Nutr Metab (Lond). 2008 Feb 20;5:6. PMID: 18289377 [PubMed - in process]

18. Mutungi G, Ratliff J, Puglisi M, Torres-Gonzalez M, Vaishnav U, Leite JO, Quann E, Volek JS, Fernandez ML., "Dietary cholesterol from eggs increases plasma HDL cholesterol in overweight men consuming a carbohydrate-restricted diet," J Nutr. 2008 Feb;138(2):272-6. PMID: 18203890 [PubMed - indexed for MEDLINE]

19. Lauheranta, A., et al. Association of the fatty acid profile of serum lipids with glucose and insulin metabolism during 2 fat-modified diets in subjects with impaired glucose tolerance. Am J Clin Nutr. 2002 Aug;76(2):331-7.

20. Romon M, Lebel P, Velly C, Marecaux N, Fruchart JC, Dallongeville J. Leptin response to carbohydrate or fat meal and association with subsequent satiety and energy intake. Institut National de la Santé et de la Recherche Médicale U-508, 59000 Lille, France

21. Di Pasquale, Mauro, B.Sc., M.D., M.R.O., M.F.S., The Anabolic Solution ™: The Definitive Metabolic Diet, Training, and Nutritional Supplement Book For Recreational And Competitive Bodybuilders

(e-book), Mauro Di Pasquale, 2002 PP 48-49

22. Peyron-Caso E, Taverna M, Guerre-Millo M, Véronèse A, Pacher N, Slama G, Rizkalla SW. "Polyunsaturated fatty acids up-regulate plasma leptin in insulin-resistant rats," J Nutr. 2002 Aug;132(8):2235-40.

23. Huang XF, Xin X, McLennan P, Storlien L., "Role of fat amount and type in ameliorating diet-induced obesity: insights at the level of hypothalamic arcuate nucleus leptin receptor, neuropeptide Y and proopiomelanocortin mRNA expression., Diabetes Obes Metab. 2004 Jan;6(1):35-44.

24. Yamada, J, et. al., "Hyperleptinemia elicited by the 5-HT precursor, 5-hydroxytryptophan in mice: involvement of insulin," Life Sci. 2003 Sep 19;73(18):2335-44.

25. Yamada, J, et. al., "Effects of insulin and adrenalectomy on elevation of serum leptin levels induced by 5-hydroxytryptophan in mice," Biol Pharm Bull. 2003 Oct;26(10):1491-3.

26. Kabir M, Guerre-Millo M, Laromiguiere M, Slama G, Rizkalla SW., "Negative regulation of leptin by chronic high-glycemic index starch diet.," Metabolism. 2000 Jun;49(6):764-9.

27. Bray, G.A., Nielsen, S.J., Popkin, B.M., "Consumption of High-Fructose Corn Syrup in Beverages May Play a Role in the Epidemic of Obesity," American Journal of Clinical Nutrition, 79(4), 2004, pages 537-543

28. Elliott SS, Keim NL, Stern JS, Teff K, Havel PJ., "Fructose, weight gain, and the insulin resistance syndrome," Am J Clin Nutr. 2002 Nov;76(5):911-22.

29. Shapiro, A., et. al., "Fructose-induced leptin resistance exacerbates weight gain in response to subsequent high-fat feeding," Am J Physiol Regul Integr Comp Physiol. 2008 Nov;295(5):R1370-5. Epub 2008 Aug 13

30. Richards, Byron J., CCN, Mastering Leptin: The Leptin Diet, Solving Obesity And Preventing Disease! (2nd edition), Minneapolis, Minnesota: Wellness Resources Books, 2002. PP 169-172

31. Richards, Byron J., CCN, Mastering Leptin: The Leptin Diet, Solv-

ing Obesity And Preventing Disease! (2nd edition), Minneapolis, Minnesota: Wellness Resources Books, 2002. PP 172-173

32. Teff, KL, et. al. "Dietary fructose reduces circulating insulin and leptin, attenuates postprandial suppression of ghrelin, and increases triglycerides in women," J Clin Endocrinol Metab. 2004 Jun;89(6):2963-72.

33. Chaudhri O, Small C, Bloom S., "Gastrointestinal hormones regulating appetite," Philos Trans R Soc Lond B Biol Sci. 2006 Jul 29;361(1471):1187-209.

34. Tannous dit El Khoury D, Obeid O, Azar ST, Hwalla N., "Variations in postprandial ghrelin status following ingestion of high-carbohydrate, high-fat, and high-protein meals in males," Ann Nutr Metab. 2006;50(3):260-9. Epub 2006 Feb 23.

35. Erdmann, J. Differential effect of protein and fat on plasma ghrelin levels in man. Regul Pept. 2003 Nov 15;116(1-3):101-7.

36. Potier M, Darcel N, Tomé D., "Protein, amino acids and the control of food intake," Curr Opin Clin Nutr Metab Care. 2009 Jan;12(1):54-8.

37. Erdmann J, Leibl M, Wagenpfeil S, Lippl F, Schusdziarra V., "Ghrelin response to protein and carbohydrate meals in relation to food intake and glycerol levels in obese subjects," Regul Pept. 2006 Jul 15;135(1-2):23-9. Epub 2006 Apr 27.

38. Sedlock DA., "The latest on carbohydrate loading: a practical approach," Curr Sports Med Rep. 2008 Jul-Aug;7(4):209-13.

39. Havemann L., et. Al., "Fat adaptation followed by carbohydrate loading compromises high-intensity sprint performance." J Appl Physiol. 2006 Jan;100(1):194-202. Epub 2005 Sep 1.

40. Burke, LM., et. al., "Adaptations to short-term high-fat diet persist during exercise despite high carbohydrate availability." Med Sci Sports Exerc. 2002 Jan;34(1):83-91.

41. Stellingwerff, T., et. Al., "Decreased PDH activation and glycogenolysis during exercise following fat adaptation with carbohydrate restoration." Am J Physiol Endocrinol Metab. 2006 Feb;290(2):E380-8. Epub 2005 Sep 27.

42. Parrish CC, Pathy DA, Angel A. Dietary fish oils limit adipose tissue hypertrophy in rats. Metabolism 1990; 39(3):217-219

43. Parrish CC, Pathy DA, Parkes JG, Angel A. Dietary fish oils modify adipocyte structure and function. Journal of Cellular Physiology 1991; 148(3):493-502

44. Harper CR, Jacobson TA. The fats of life: the role of omega-3 fatty acids in the prevention of coronary heart disease. Arch Intern Med. 2001 Oct 8;161(18):2185-92.

45. Durrington PN, Bhatnagar D, Mackness MI, Morgan J, Julier K, Khan MA, France M. An omega-3 polyunsaturated fatty acid concentrate administered for one year decreased triglycerides in simvastatin treated patients with coronary heart disease and persisting hypertriglyceridaemia. Heart. 2001 May;85(5):544-8.

46. Nordoy A, Marchioli R, Arnesen H, Videbaek J. n-3 polyunsaturated fatty acids and cardiovascular diseases. Lipids. 2001;36 Suppl:S127-9.

47. Engler MM, Engler MB, Pierson DM, Molteni LB, Molteni A Effects of docosahexaenoic acid on vascular pathology and reactivity in hypertension. Exp Biol Med (Maywood). 2003 Mar;228(3):299-307.

48. Passfall J, Philipp T, Woermann F, Quass P, Thiede M, Haller H. Different effects of eicosapentaenoic acid and olive oil on blood pressure, intracellular free platelet calcium, and plasma lipids in patients with essential hypertension. Clin Investig. 1993 Aug;71(8):628-33.

49. Bhatnagar D, Durrington PN.Omega-3 fatty acids: their role in the prevention and treatment of atherosclerosis related risk factors and complications. Int J Clin Pract. 2003 May;57(4):305-14

50. Holm T, Andreassen AK, Aukrusst P, Andersen K, Geiran OR, Kjekshus J, Simonsen S, Gullestad L. Omega-3 fatty acids improve blood pressure control and preserve renal function in hypertensive heart transplant recipients. Eur Heart J. 2001 Mar;22(5):428-36.

51. Donadio JV. n-3 Fatty acids and their role in nephrologic practice. Curr Opin Nephrol Hypertens. 2001 Sep;10(5):639-42.

52. Vergili-Nelsen JM. Benefits of fish oil supplementation for hemodialysis patients. J Am Diet Assoc. 2003 Sep;103(9):1174-7.

53. Atkins, Robert C., M.D., Dr. Atkins' Vita-Nutrient Solution: Nature's Answer To Drugs, Fireside, 1999. Page 209

Sixth Prescription: Eat the Foods That Heal, Avoid the Foods That Kill

1. Rankin, J.W., "Role of Protein in Exercise," Clin Sports Med 18.3 (1999) : 499-511.

2. Boirie, Y., et al., "Slow and Fast Dietary Proteins Differently Modulate Postprandial Protein Accretion," Proc Natl Acad Sci U S A 94.26 (1997) : 14930-5.

3. Gaudichon, C., et al., "Net Postprandial Utilization of (15N)-Labeled Milk Protein Nitrogen Is Influenced by Diet Composition in Humans," J Nutr 129.4 (1999) : 890-5.

4. Poortmans, J.R., and Dellalieux, O., "Do regular high protein diets have potential health risks on kidney function in athletes?" International Journal of Sports Nutrition and Exercise Metabolism, 10:28-38, 2000.

5. Edelman, Steven V., M.D., et al, Taking Control Of Your Diabetes (2nd Edition), Professional Communications Inc., 2001. PP 58-60

6. Giacco, R., et al. Dietary fibre in treatment of diabetes: myth or reality? Dig Liver Dis. 2002 Sep;34 Suppl 2:S140-4.

7. Ou, S. In vitro study of possible role of dietary fiber in lowering postprandial serum glucose. J Agric Food Chem. 2001 Feb;49(2):1026-9.

8. Miles, C., et al. Effect of dietary fiber on the metabolizable energy of human diets. J Nutr 1988 Sep;118(9):1075-81.

9. Holt, S., et al. A satiety index of common foods. Eur J Clin Nutr. 1995 Sep;49(9):675-90.

10. Terpstra, A.H., Javadi, M., Beynen, A.C., et al., "Dietary conjugated linoleic acids as free fatty acids and triaglycerols similarly affect body composition and energy balance in mice," Journal of Nutrition, 133:3181-3186, 2003.

11. Gittleman, Ann Louise, M.S., C.N.S., The Fat Flush Plan, McGraw Hill, 2002. PP30-31

12. Atkins, Robert C., M.D., Dr. Atkins' Vita-Nutrient Solution: Nature's Answer To Drugs, Fireside, 1999. PP 225-227

13. Forsythe, Casandra, M.S., Women's Health Perfect Body Diet: The Ultimate Weight Loss And Workout Plan To Drop Stubborn Pounds And Get Fit For Life!, Rodale, 2008. PP 32, 37, 91

14. Gittleman, Ann Louise, M.S., C.N.S., The Fat Flush Plan, McGraw Hill, 2002. Page 6

15. Forsythe, Casandra, M.S., Women's Health Perfect Body Diet: The Ultimate Weight Loss And Workout Plan To Drop Stubborn Pounds And Get Fit For Life!, Rodale, 2008. PP 58-59

Seventh Prescription: Choose Your Carbs Wisely

1. Spiller, G.A., Jensen, C.D., Pattison, T.S., et al., "Effect of protein dose on serum glucose and insulin response to sugars," American Journal of Clinical Nutrition, 46:474-481, 1987

2. Kohler, John, "The Truth about Agave Syrup: Not as Healthy as You May Think," http://www.living-foods.com/articles/agave.html. Accessed on 11/7/2009.

3. Glucerna Website, http://glucerna.com/product/snackshakes.aspx. Accessed on 11/7/2009.

4. http://www.glycemicindex.com. Accessed on 11/7/2009.

5. Edelman, Steven V., M.D., et al, Taking Control Of Your Diabetes (2nd Edition), Professional Communications Inc., 2001, pages 130-132

6. Korenman, Stanley G., Kahn, C. Ronald, Atlas of Clinical Endocrinology, Volume 2: Diabetes, Bristol-Myers Squibb, 2000, page 9

7. Gerich, John E., "Is Reduced First-Phase Insulin Release the Earliest Detectable Abnormality in Individuals Destined to Develop Type II Diabetes?" accessed from http://diabetes.diabetesjournals.org/cgi/content/full/51/suppl_1/S117 on 3-3-2009.

8. Heath, J., "Maximizing Nutrient Partitioning: The Insulin Myth" http://www.figureathlete.com/free_online_article/diet_and_nutrition/maximizing_nutrient_partitioning_the_insulin_myth, first ac-

cessed December 1st, 2008

9. Sigal RJ, El-Hashimy M, Martin BC, Soeldner JS, Krolewski AS, Warram JH. "Acute postchallenge hyperinsulinemia predicts weight gain: a prospective study," .Diabetes. 1997 Jun;46(6):1025-9

10. Schwartz MW, Boyko EJ, Kahn SE, Ravussin E, Bogardus C., "Reduced insulin secretion: an independent predictor of body weight gain," J Clin Endocrinol Metab. 1995 May;80(5):1571-6.

11. SH Holt, JC Miller, and P Petocz, An insulin index of foods: the insulin demand generated by 1000-kJ portions of common foods, Am J Clin Nutr 1997 66: 1264-1276 Am J Clin Nutr PubMed abstract

12. http://www.mendosa.com/insulin_index.htm

13. Holt, S., et al. A satiety index of common foods. Eur J Clin Nutr. 1995 Sep;49(9):675-90.

14. Kissileff, H. The satiating efficiency of foods. Physiol Behav. 1984 Feb;32(2):319-32.

15. Editors, Alcohol search done at http://www.nutritiondata.com, accessed 3-4-2009.

Eighth Prescription:
Know What, When, and How Much to Eat

1. Shah M, Miller DS, Geissler CA,."Lower metabolic rates of post-obese versus lean women: thermogenesis, basal metabolic rate and genetics," Eur J Clin Nutr. 1988 Sep; 42(9):741-52.

2. Bessard T, Schutz Y, Jéquier E., "Energy expenditure and postprandial thermogenesis in obese women before and after weight loss," Am J Clin Nutr. 1983 Nov; 38(5):680-93.

3. Leibel RL, Rosenbaum M, Hirsch J, "Changes in energy expenditure resulting from altered body weight," N Engl J Med. 1995 Mar 9; 332(10):621-8.

4. Rosenbaum, M, Hirsch, J, Gallagher, DA, Leibel, RL, "Long-term persistence of adaptive thermogenesis in subjects who have maintained a reduced body weight," Am J Clin Nutr, 2008 Oct; 88(4):906-12.

5. Weigle DS, Sande KJ, Iverius PH, Monsen ER, Brunzell JD, "Weight

loss leads to a marked decrease in nonresting energy expenditure in ambulatory human subjects," Metabolism. 1988 Oct; 37(10):930-6.

6. Levine, J.A., et. al., "Role of nonexercise activity thermogenesis in resistance to fat gain in humans Science," Volume 283, Issue 5399 (8 January 1999), 212-214

7. Wang et. al. "Brain dopamine and obesity," The Lancet. Volume 357, Issue 9253, 3 February 2001, Pages 354-357

8. Forbes, G.B. "Body fat content influences the body composition response to nutrition and exercise," Annual New York Academy of Science, 904 (2000) 359-65.

9. Dulloo, A.G.; Jacquet J., "The control of partitioning between protein and fat during human starvation: its internal determinants and biological significance," British Journal of Nutrition, 82 (1999), 339-356

10. Dulloo, A.G. "Partitioning between protein and fat during starvation and refeeding: is the assumption of intra-individual constancy of P-ratio valid?" British Journal of Nutrition, 79 (1998), 107-113

11. Frankenfield DC, Muth ER, Rowe WA., "The Harris-Benedict studies of human basal metabolism: history and limitations," J Am Diet Assoc. 1998 Apr; 98(4):439-45.

12. Dobratz JR, Sibley SD, Beckman TR, Valentine BJ, Kellogg TA, Ikramuddin S, Earthman CP., "Predicting energy expenditure in extremely obese women," JPEN J Parenter Enteral Nutr. 2007 May-Jun; 31(3):217-27.

13. Lazzer S, Agosti F, Resnik M, Marazzi N, Mornati D, Sartorio A. "Prediction of resting energy expenditure in severely obese Italian males." J Endocrinol Invest. 2007 Oct;30(9):754-61.

14. Lazzer S, Agosti F, Silvestri P, Derumeaux-Burel H, Sartorio A." Prediction of resting energy expenditure in severely obese Italian women.," J Endocrinol Invest. 2007 Jan;30(1):20-7.

15. Weijs PJ., "Validity of predictive equations for resting energy expenditure in US and Dutch overweight and obese class I and II adults aged 18-65 y," Am J Clin Nutr;88(4):959-70, 2008 Oct.

16. Mifflin MD, St Jeor ST, Hill LA, Scott BJ, Daugherty SA, Koh YO.

"A new predictive equation for resting energy expenditure in healthy individuals.", Am J Clin Nutr., 1990 Feb;51(2):241-7. PMID: 2305711

17. Frankenfield D, Roth-Yousey L, Compher C. "Comparison of predictive equations for resting metabolic rate in healthy nonobese and obese adults: a systematic review," J Am Diet Assoc. 2005 May;105(5):775-89.

18. Johnston CS, Day CS, Swan PD., "Postprandial thermogenesis is increased 100% on a high-protein, low-fat diet versus a high-carbohydrate, low-fat diet in healthy, young women," J Am Coll Nutr. 2002 Feb;21(1):55-61.

19. Speechly, D. and Buffenstein, R. Greater appetite control associated with an increased frequency of eating in lean males. Appetite 1999 33(3): 285-297.

20. Jenkins, D., et al. Nibbling versus gorging: metabolic advantages of increased meal frequency. N Engl J Med 1989 321(14): 929-934.

21. Rosenbaum M, et. al., "Low-dose leptin reverses skeletal muscle, autonomic, and neuroendocrine adaptations to maintenance of reduced weight," J. Clin. Invest. 115(12): 3579-3586 (2005).

22. deCastro, J. (1987). Circadian rhythms of the spontaneous meal pattern, macronutrient intake, and mood of humans. Physiol Behav 40(4): 437-446.

23. Wu, M., et al. (1986). Diurnal variation of insulin clearance and sensitivity n normal man. Prc Natl Sci Counc Repub China B 10(1): 64-69.

24. JVerrillo A, De Teresa A, Martino C, et al. Differential roles of splanchnic and peripheral tissues in determining diurnal fluctuation of glucose tolerance. Am J Physiol 1989; 257(4 pt 1):E459.

25. Berardi, John, "G-Flux: Building The Ultimate Body," http://www.t-nation.com/free_online_article/sports_body_training_performance_nutrition/gflux_building_the_ultimate_body, accessed 11-23-2008

Ninth Prescription:
Know Your Diabetic Complications, Their Medications, and Your Alternatives

1. Gittleman, Ann Louise, M.S., C.N.S., The Fat Flush Plan, McGraw Hill, 2002. Pages 4-5 & 17-18

2. Edelman, Steven V., M.D., et al, Taking Control Of Your Diabetes (2nd Edition), Professional Communications Inc., 2001. Pages 103-119

3. Vernon, M., Eberstein, J., Atkins Diabetes Revolution (1st Edition) New York: Harper Collins, 2004, Page 78-83 & 475-479

4. Atkins, Robert C., M.D., Dr. Atkins' New Diet Revolution, M. Evans and Company, Inc., 2002, PP 224-233

5. McCarty, M.F., "The Case for Supplemental Chromium and a Survey of Clinical Studies with Chromium Picolinate," J Appl Nutr 43 (1991) : 59-66.

6. Mertz, W., "Interaction of Chromium with Insulin: A Progress Report," Nutr Rev 56.6 (1998) : 174-7.

7. Riales, R., and Albrink, M.J., "Effect of Chromium Chloride Supplementation on Glucose Tolerance and Serum Lipids Including High-Density Lipoprotein of Adult Men," Am J Clin Nutr 34.12 (1981) : 2670-78.

8. Goldfine AB, Patti ME, Zuberi L, Goldstein BJ, LeBlanc R, Landaker EJ, Jiang ZY, Willsky GR, Kahn CR. "Metabolic effects of vanadyl sulfate in humans with non insulin dependent diabetes mellitus: in vivo and vitro studies." Metabolsim 2000 Mar; 49(3):400-10

9. Goldfine, A.B., et al., "Metabolic Effects of Vanadyl Sulfate in Humans with Non-Insulin-Dependent Diabetes Mellitus: In Vivo and In Vitro Studies," Metabolism 49.3 (2000) : 400-10.

10. Kelly, G.S., "Insulin Resistance: Lifestyle and Nutritional Interventions," Altern Med Rev 5.2 (2000) : 109-32.

11. Editors at Nutros.Com (Chromium), http://nutros.com/nsr-0201p. html, accessed on 1-14-2009

12. Editors at Nutros.Com (Vanadium), http://nutros.com/nsr-0203h. html, accessed on 1-14-2009

13. Angelico, M., et al., "Improvement in Serum Lipid Profile in Hyper-Lipoproteinaemic Patients After Treatment with Pantethine: A Crossover, Double-Blind Trial Versus Placebo," Curr Ther Res 33 (1983) : 1091.

14. Bertolini, S., et al., "Lipoprotein Changes Induced by Pantethine in Hyperlipoproteinemic Patients: Adults and Children," Int J Clin Pharmacol Ther Toxicol 24 (1986) : 630-7.

15. Fidanza, A., "Therapeutic Action of Pantothenic Acid," Int J Vitam Nutr Res Suppl 24 (1983) : 53-67.

16. Gaddi, A., et al., "Controlled Evaluation of Pantethine, a Natural Hypolipidemic Compound, in Patients with Different Forms of Hyperlipoproteinemia," Atherosclerosis 50 (1984) : 73-83.

17. Atkins, Robert C., M.D., Dr. Atkins' Vita-Nutrient Solution: Nature's Answer To Drugs, Fireside, 1999. Page 84

18. Jacob S, Rnus P, Hermann R, Tritschler HJ, Maerker E, Renn W, Augustin HJ, Dietze GJ, Rett K. "Oral administration of RAE-ALA modulates insulin sensitivity in patients with type II diabetes mellitus: a placebo controlled pilot trial." Free Radic Biol Med 1999 Aug; 27(3-4):309-

19. Jacob S, Henriksen EJ, Schiemann AL, Simon I, Clancy DE, Tritschler HJ, Jung WI, Augustin HJ, Dietze GJ. "Enhancement of glucose disposal in patients with type II diabetes by ALA." Arzneimittel forschung 1995 Aug;45(8):872-4

20. Atkins, Robert C., M.D., Dr. Atkins' Vita-Nutrient Solution: Nature's Answer To Drugs, Fireside, 1999. Page 252

21. Editors at Nutros.Com (Alpha Lipoic Acid), http://nutros.com/nsr-0202i.html, accessed on 1-14-2009

22. NaKaya Y, Minami A, Harada N, Sakamoto S, Niwa Y, Ohnaka M. "Taurine improves insulin sensitivity in the Otsuka Long-Evans Tokushima fatty rat, a model of spontaneous type II diabetes. Am J Clin Nutr 2000 Jan; 71(1):54-8

23. Militante, J.D., Lombardini, J. B., "Treatment of Hypertension with Oral Taurine: Experimental and Clinical Studies," Amino Acids, 23(4), 2002, PP381-393

24. Atkins, Robert C., M.D., Dr. Atkins' Vita-Nutrient Solution: Nature's Answer To Drugs, Fireside, 1999. Pages 184-187

25. Editors at Nutros.Com (Taurine), http://nutros.com/nsr-02015.html, accessed on 1-14-2009

26. G. Paolisso et al., "Chronic Intake of Pharmacological Doses of vitamin E Might be Useful in the Therapy of Elderly Patients with Coronary Heart Disease." Am. J Clin Nutr 61(1995):848-52

27. Rosolova H, Mayer O Jr., Reaven GM. "Insulin-mediated glucose disposal is decreased in normal subjects with relatively low plasma magnesium concentrations." Metabolism 2000 Mar;49(3):418-20

28. Barbagallo M, Dominguez LJ, Tagliamonte MR, Resnick LM, Paolisso G. "Effects of vitamin E and glutathione on glucose metabolism: role of magnesium." Hypertension 1999 Oct;34(4pt2):1002-6

29. Kawano, Y., et al., "Effects of Magnesium Supplementation in Hypertensive Patients: Assessment by Office, Home, and Ambulatory Blood Pressures," Hypertension 32.2 (1998) : 260-5.

30. Rude, R., Manoogian, C., Ehlrich, L., et. al., "Mechanisms of Blood Pressure Regulation by Magnesium in Man," Magnesium, 8(5-6), 1989, PP 266-273.

31. Editors at Nutros.Com (Magnesium), http://nutros.com/nsr-02023.html, accessed on 1-14-2009

32. Editors at Nutros.Com (Calcium), http://nutros.com/nsr-020lj.html, accessed on 1-14-2009

33. Fujioka, T., et al., "Clinical Study of Cardiac Arrhythmias Using a 24-Hour Continuous Electrocardiographic Recorder (5th Report)- Antiarrhythmic Action of Coenzyme Q10 in Diabetics," Tohoku J Exp Med 141S(1983) : 453-63.

34. Kamikawa, T., et al., "Effects of Coenzyme Q10 on Exercise Tolerance in Chronic Stable Angina Pectoris," Am J Cardiol 56.4 (1985) : 247-51.

35. Morisco, C., et al., "Effect of Coenzyme Q10 Therapy in Patients with Congestive Heart Failure: A Long-Term Multicenter Randomized Study," Clin Investig 71.85 (1993) : S134-6.

36. Mortensen, S.A., et al., "Long-Term Coenzyme Q10 Therapy: A Ma-

jor Advance in the Management of Resistant Myocardial Failure," Drug Exp Clin Res 11.8 (1985) : 581-93.

37. Murray, M.T., Encyclopedia of Nutritional Supplements (Prima Publishing, Rocklin, CA, 1996) 296-308.

38. Singh, R.B., et al., "Effect of Hydrosoluble Coenzyme Q10 on Blood Pressures and Insulin Resistance in Hypertensive Patients with Coronary Artery Disease," J Hum Hypertens 13.3 (1999) : 203-8.

39. Tanaka, J., et al., "Coenzymed Q10: The Prophylactic Effect on Low Cardiac Output Following Cardiac Valve Replacement," Ann Thorac Surg 33.2 (1982) : 145-51.

40. Editors at Nutros.Com (Carnitine), http://nutros.com/nsr-0201k.html, accessed on 1-14-2009

41. Pola, P., et al., "Carnitine in the Therapy of Dyslipidemic Patients," Curr Ther Res Clin Exp 27.2 (1980) : 208-216.

42. Pola, P., et al., "Statistical Evaluation of Long-Term L-Carnitine Therapy in Hyper-Lipo Proteinemias," Drugs Exp Clin Res 9.12 (1983) : 925-934.

43. Editors at Nutros.Com (CoQ10), http://nutros.com/nsr-0201q.html, accessed on 1-14-2009

44. Atkins, Robert C., M.D., Dr. Atkins' Vita-Nutrient Solution: Nature's Answer To Drugs, Fireside, 1999. Pages 80 & 90

45. Cressey, E., "Fish Advice, Part I," http://ericcressey.com/fishy-advice-part-I, accessed 6-01-2008

46. Atkins, Robert C., M.D., Dr. Atkins' Vita-Nutrient Solution: Nature's Answer To Drugs, Fireside, 1999. Pages 216-221

47. Imai, K., and Nakachi, K., "Cross Sectional Study of Effects of Drinking Green Tea on Cardiovascular and Liver Diseases (see comments)," BMJ 310.6981 (1995) : 693-6.

INDEX

CONELY BRANCH